KU-686-983

WITHDRAWN

Contents

Expert Advisory Panel

We are extremely grateful to the following people – all of whom are top experts in their fields – for their help, professional advice and enthusiasm with the book:

Professor Felicity Reynolds, Professor of Obstetric Anaesthesia (the only one in the UK) at St Thomas's Hospital, London

Dr David Bogod, Consultant Obstetric Anaesthetist at Nottingham City Hospital, and Secretary of the Obstetric Anaesthetists Association

Dr Christopher Wells, Director of the Pain Research Unit at the Walton Hospital in Liverpool

Rowena Davies, Head of Midwifery Services at St George's Hospital. Also the entire midwifery and community midwife team there, especially Lilian Meeran and Narinda Cooper

Professor Richard Cooke, President of the British Society of Perinatal Medicine

Professor Nicholas Fisk of the Institute of Obstetrics at Queen Charlotte's Hospital, London

Acupuncture: Christina McCausland, acupuncturist and co-founder of Acupuncture for Childbirth

Water: Janet Balaskas, founder of the Active Birth Movement and Dr Yehudi Gordon, the St John and St Elisabeth/Royal Garden Hospitals, London

Aromatherapy: Dr Vivienne Lunny, former pathologist and now Head of Research for the Aromatherapy Organizations Council's scientific committee

Homeopathy: Barbara Cummins, homeopath and midwife

The Royal College of Midwives, especially their President, independent midwife Caroline Flint (also founder of the Birth Centre, London) and Melanie Every, Head of Professional Training

Autogenic Training: Dr Alice Green, homeopath, diploma in obstetrics and Vice President of the British Autogenic Training Association

Hypnotherapy: Dr Les Brann, GP and hypnotherapist, who works with the Chelmsford Hospital training women in antenatal self-hypnosis

Massage: Stephen Sandler, Director of the Expectant Mothers Clinic at the British School of Osteopathy; also consultant osteopath at the Portland Hospital for Women & Children in London

Breathing and Relaxation: Helen Lewison, at the time of writing Chairwoman of the National Childbirth Trust

Professor Michael Chapman, former Head of Obstetrics & Gynaecology at Guy's Hospital, London, now has the same title at St George's Hospital, Sydney, Australia

Breast Pain: Hilary Idzikowska, Research Collator for the La Leche League of Great Britain

Sheila Tunstall, Information Co-ordinator of the Caesarean Support Network

Beverley Beech, Chairwoman of the Association for Improvement of Midwifery Services

Reflexology: Fara Begum Baig, PhD in Biochemistry, teaches reflexology to the doctors, nurses and midwives of Addenbrookes Hospital, Cambridge and at Ely Hospital, both as stress control and for obstetric purposes. Also director of the Hope Street Holistic Centre in Cambridge

Professor Peter Hepper, Head of the Psychology Department at Queen's University, Belfast

Dr Lennart Righard, Consultant in Paediatrics at Malmo General Hospital and the University of Lund, Sweden

Introduction

The sight of 70,000 words on pain relief in labour may – initially – be thoroughly daunting. Enough to make any woman wonder if perhaps pain is all there is to childbirth. And does it really hurt *that* much?

The good news is that the answer to both questions is No. And even if it does hurt there's plenty that you, your partner, your midwife and doctor can do to ensure that it does not hurt badly for long. Further, some labours either *are* virtually painless, or can be made so with good analgesia.

The fact that most women do, quite voluntarily, go through labour more than once, also confirms that any labour pain is unlike ordinary pain, and therefore far easier to cope with. Everyday pain is when you accidentally shut your finger in a door. This hurts instantly, and constantly. Labour contraction pain behaves very differently because it:

- Begins slowly and gently, builds to a climax, then recedes. There is a rest in between times of anything from half an hour, if you are in early labour, to a minute or two if you are near to giving birth to your baby, when you can get your breath back.

- Labour pain can almost always be, to a great extent, either relieved or coped with. Sometimes it can be obliterated altogether.

- Everyone's experience of labour is different – as different as the women and their babies themselves. Some are very short and virtually pain-free, over within an hour. Others may be long and difficult. Most are somewhere in between.

- Mothers often also say they found they could handle the sensations they experienced in their labours just fine. For some, this may be because they had been worried about the idea of childbirth, but when it was actually happening they found it was not nearly as bad as they had feared. Many say it was because they were able to find within themselves deep resources of calm, strength and natural coping ability which they never imagined they had.

However, some midwives and medical staff don't always explain these things, and neither do many other women who have had babies. Some of them say this is because the pregnant woman simply never asked them. This may well be true, as most have a quiet, instinctive and generally well-justified confidence that they will be able to manage their own labours perfectly well.

Others claim they did answer pregnant women's questions about what to expect in childbirth but that they had a feeling their audience was not quite taking it in. This might also have an element of truth in it. The enormous hormonal changes of pregnancy can make absorbing new, detailed information difficult. Many women report that towards the end of their pregnancies they felt they had simply switched off mentally for a while, and that things they would usually have worried about did not seem to be able to reach them. Some say they felt like this all the way through, as if their pregnancy was insulating them from the rest of the world.

But this is not the whole story. There is still a slight sense of a well-meaning but ultimately unhelpful attitude that 'We don't want to frighten first-timers.' Or 'If we tell her too much about it she'll only go away and worry,' when those who know something about it should be sharing their knowledge and experience. This would give pregnant women the opportunity to prepare themselves for their own labours, if they wanted to, in whatever ways they feel would help them the most. It would also give them the time to consider the pros and cons of the different pain-relief methods and coping strategies.

The result is that many women who are pregnant for the first time are left with the distinct impression that pain control is a relatively minor consideration and that it doesn't much matter what sort you have – if any. Some may also be given to understand that they might experience some 'discomfort' (a traditional euphemism for childbirth pain) but that is all. Full throttle labour is not a good time to discover that you have been misled.

At the other end of the scale are women who have been so scared by alarming stories from other mothers ('What I went through') that they have had all their natural confidence eroded and end up frightened that they will not be able to cope with the reportedly awful pain of it all. 'My first was over 10lbs. She took three days and I had 94 stitches. You look like you're having a really big one too – it's in the family, you know,' said my usually kindly mother-in-law as I neared the end of my first pregnancy. Scared out of my wits, I went straight to my obstetrician and begged to pay for a caesarean. When Ben finally arrived – vaginally – he was all of 6lbs 13 oz.

Having spoken to literally hundreds of women who have had babies, the vast majority of them do say that the birth of their child was the most astounding, moving and important experience they had ever had. And for most, it seemed to make no difference, from the point of view of sheer wonder and the feeling that it had all been worth it, whether they had had an easy birth or a more difficult one. Many said they positively enjoyed some parts of labour and giving birth, were fascinated by other parts and could put up with the rest (on the understanding that it wouldn't last long). Almost all added that there were also certain periods they had just wanted to be over.

Perhaps it is partly these contrasts, together with each woman's natural ability to give birth in her own way, which makes childbirth so extraordinary. And so special.

This book sets out to explore the pros and cons of *all* possible pain-relief options, so that you can make the most informed decision possible about what's best for *you*. And to ensure that you have access to the pain-relief method you feel will suit you best. Knowledge is power. It also drives out fear.

Nikki Bradford
1995

Preparation

'Getting into training for childbirth is like training to run the London marathon,' says Steven Sandler, Director of the Expectant Mothers Clinic at the British School of Osteopathy, and father of three. 'Both are major, sustained physical efforts with people cheering you on, a huge hormonal buzz, and a tremendous feeling of exhilaration, satisfaction and delight at the end. With preparation, knowledge and training you're a winner. Without, and you'll probably only get halfway round before collapsing with exhaustion.'

Childbirth preparation classes, whether they are run by your local hospital or health centre, or privately by the NCT or Active Birth teachers, are invaluable here. But they do not always tell you everything you need to know about *all* the possible pain-relief options as there is a lot of other ground to cover as well, and often there simply isn't the time to go over it all in detail – which is where this book can help you.

Finding out as much as possible about pain-relief options so you have all the information you need when you want it is a vital part of preparation for childbirth. But you may need to start early – at least by the time you are two-thirds of the way through your pregancy.

This is because many of the natural methods either need you to practise them for a few weeks to get maximum benefit (self-hypnosis, pp. 169–78), breathing and relaxation (pp. 126–37), visualization (pp. 134–7), or you need to find practitioners who can familiarize you with the therapy you would like to use (homeopathy, pp. 160–69, acupuncture, pp. 137–44, aromatherapy, pp. 144–53). These therapists will often provide you with a customized birth kit of their remedies, and some techniques you can use yourself – for instance, specific acupressure points to press, particular aromatherapy oils to massage into your skin or homeopathic remedies to take at different stages, in varying circumstances.

Many of these therapists also advocate a few full treatments from mid- to late pregnancy, all of which takes time. Other methods, such as immersion in a birthing pool of water may take some arranging (see pp. 178–88), from the point of view of finding a hospital which has one, or which will allow you to bring your own, then hiring the pool, setting it up, etc). If you would like to have a complementary therapist with you in labour, if you are having a hospital birth you need to be sure that the hospital is happy about this – and if not, either take time to argue your case or find another unit which raises no objections (see pp. 9, 124–5, 202–3).

A bit of research can pay dividends where pharmacological methods are concerned too. For instance, if you are interested in having Entonox as an option, the middle of labour is not a good time to discover that the smell makes you feel sick, so try it out first during one of your antenatal visits to the hospital. If you are having a home birth, ask the midwife looking after you whether you can try it out at home or at the antenatal clinic.

If you feel an epidural would suit you best, check that the hospital has 24-hour anaesthetist cover for this. The smaller hospitals tend not to, and this may mean that on the day (or night) you might not be able to have the pain relief you had been banking on to help you, and this can be a devastating discovery if your labour is proving painful (see pp. 75–90). If you are interested in the mood enhancement and relaxation that pethidine can offer but are worried it could make your baby sleepy, discuss with the midwives what dosage they use, and when, at one of your routine antenatal appointments. You might also want to call one of the childbirth help organizations such as AIMS (see **Resources**) to see how best pethidine may be used (see pp. 106–13).

Potential pain and discomfort after labour is an area which women tend to get little information on until they are experiencing it (see pp. 215–19), but again some pre-planning can be very helpful indeed. For instance, there are many ways to try and minimize the likelihood of your needing an episiotomy or tear (see pp. 7–10, 272–81); comforting herbal solutions which can be prepared for use at home or in hospital which may speed healing of the perineal and vulval areas (see p. 227); and homeopathic preparations said to reduce bruising and to encourage healing (see pp. 7, 160). All these are worth checking out before you actually need to use them.

Another important part of preparation for labour as a whole, and for the type of pain relief you feel would suit you best during it, is making a birth plan. But try to include a section on after the birth too. Very few women do this, as the labour itself tends to be at the forefront of everyone's mind. Yet what happens afterwards and how it is managed can be as important as the childbirth itself from the point of view of the comfort and well-being of you and your baby (see pp. 7–10).

Homeopathic treatments

Taken before and during the birth, remedies such as Arnica (see **Homeopathy** pp. 160–69) are said to help reduce bruising, swelling and inflammation which can make an episiotomy site so sore afterwards.

MAKING A BIRTHPLAN

This is a good way of communicating your wishes *in writing* so they can be attached to your medical notes for future reference. It can also help you sort out in your own mind what you feel is important and what you would – or would not – be happy with. Keep a copy and take it with you if you are going to hospital to have your baby so that you or your partner can then refer the staff to it if necessary.

About 10 to 15 per cent of women do make birthplans, but most concentrate solely on the delivery and labour. Yet the time immediately afterward is also very important, so try to decide what you would like to happen then as well, to give both you and your baby the peace and calm to recover and get to know each other.

It may help to speak to your local childbirthing group (see **Resources**) or community midwife about the sort of things to consider covering in the plan, but the following are some of the points that you may want to include (pain relief is only one element):

1. People: Who is going to be there at the birth apart from the midwife – your partner, a friend, your mother? Would you object to midwifery or medical students watching or helping you?

2. Medical interventions: What are your feelings about episiotomy, forceps or ventouse delivery, acceleration of labour, caesarean section? All are commonly performed in labour. They can be vital life-saving procedures, but some maternity units are quicker to do them than others. All involve additional discomfort/pain.

For instance, a labour which is accelerated with a drip tends to mean sharper contractions, far closer together, all the way through the birth process. They will not build up gently but come on with their full force each time. This makes them harder to cope with than natural labour contractions which tend to start gently, build up to a peak then die away, giving you a rest of between twenty minutes in early labour or two or three minute in late labour to recover between each one, and only become really painful and close together for the last hour or so. This is why many women decide to have an epidural with an accelerated labour.

Which interventions would you want to avoid if at all possible, and which might you have no especial objection to?

3. Pain Relief: What would you prefer to use – in order of preference? What facilities does the hospital, if that is where you are having your baby, offer? Twenty-four hour epidural cover? Several TENS machines? A water pool? If they do not offer the method of your choice, what do they feel about you bringing equipment with you, such as a hired water pool or TENS machine, a borrowed birth cushion, a hypnotherapy tape and tape recorder? If you want a complementary therapy which involves the presence of a trained therapist, is the hospital happy about this? And if not, who do you need to discuss it with?

4. Monitoring and Examinations: How do you feel about any monitoring of the baby (fetal monitoring), and the different techniques used?

What about internal examinations for you yourself, which the medical staff will want to carry out at intervals to check how far your cervix has dilated? Many women say these are very uncomfortable if carried out while you are lying flat on your back with your knees raised. It may be more comfortable to have them done as you lie on your side. Or ask if they can be done with you standing, perhaps with one leg raised on a chair, if you are going to be moving about upright a lot anyway.

5. Positions for labour and birth: Would you be allowed to move around as much as you want, or to give birth in a particular position if there is no medical reason why you shouldn't?

6. Your surroundings: Would you prefer to be able to dim the lights, have music playing quietly, bring in your own beanbag and cushions to lean over? Is this all right by the hospital – do they have enough room, or will you be in labour on a ward with only a little space around the bed, separated from your neighbours by curtains?

7. Who do you want to deliver your baby and carry out any stitching which might be necessary afterwards: A midwife? Doctor? Would you object to a trainee under supervision?

8. After your baby is born: Do you want the umbilical cord cut only when it has stopped pulsating? Have you any feelings about an injection to speed up the placenta's delivery? Would you prefer your baby to be put into your arms straight away before any checking of its reflexes, cleaning or weighing are carried out? Do you want to try and breastfeed him or her straight away?

Be prepared to be flexible if necessary. A birthplan represents what you would *ideally* like, if everything goes smoothly at the birth. If it doesn't you may need to change your plan – or part of it – accordingly.

WHAT HAPPENS IN LABOUR

The Labour Process

WAITING FOR LABOUR TO START

Towards the very end of their pregnancies, most women begin to feel as if they have definitely had enough. They are likely to be growing increasingly uncomfortable because of their expanding shape and size. And mothers who have developed pregnancy problems such as backache, tiredness, piles or varicose veins will probably find these get worse as the weeks go by.

The popular image of a very pregnant woman is someone who is glowing with calm and contentment over her rounded but neat belly. In reality, many will find that their abdomen has apparently dropped down to their knees and the baby's firmly engaged head is making walking uncomfortable, leaving them counting the days until their delivery date.

But only an estimated 5 per cent of babies arrive on the date their mother was given early in pregnancy. This date is intended only as a guide, with about two weeks' leeway on either side.

An expected delivery date (in clinical shorthand on all maternity forms you will see it written as EDD) is a mathematical probability based on the pregnancies of a large number of women whose expected delivery dates have been calculated on the basis of the first day of their last regular menstrual period. This calculation should only be used for women who have a 28-day cycle, as it assumes ovulation has taken place exactly halfway through it on day 14.

However, these calculations are seldom very accurate because:

Only about 8 per cent of women really do have a 28-day cycle. The others have cycles which are shorter, say 25 to 26 days, or longer, 30 to 35 days.

Ovulation day tends to move around a bit as it is affected by several different factors, from illness and stress to jet lag. Sometimes it may fall right in the middle on day 14, sometimes in the first week, sometimes in their third week. There have been cases of women ovulating a day or two after their period finished, and of women getting pregnant when they had unprotected sex while menstruating.

Not all babies stay in the womb for 40 weeks. Even when women have been very sure of their date of conception, some babies seem to prefer to stay where they are for another week or two, others are apparently ready to be born sooner, arriving a couple of weeks early.

Scans of the baby are often more help in estimating the date; based on its size and development it is possible to work out its age in the womb. But even scans are not always accurate, despite the fact that the technology used is becoming increasingly sophisticated.

It is also possible to go into premature labour before the baby is physiologically ready. Twins and triplets have a higher probability of premature arrival than a single baby. Other causes include illness (such as pre-eclampsia), shock, trauma, or prolonged stress in the mother. During the civil war in Bosnia, British charity medical workers reported that many more babies were born prematurely.

About 90 per cent of babies are born between 38 and 41 weeks after the first day of their mother's last menstrual period. About 4 per cent are born late, defined as after 42 weeks. Some 6 per cent are born early, that is before 38 weeks. All these arrival zones can be perfectly normal.

Your delivery day date is a guide, not an absolute – and as such, is likely to pass without incident. It may be more helpful to have in mind an expected delivery zone – a week or even fortnight, instead.

LABOUR

Labour generally lasts for anything between 6 and 24 hours. However, the average is longer for first births (7–9 hours) and shorter for subsequent births (4–5 hours). It consists of three main (some would argue four) stages:

The first stage involves muscle contractions of your womb as it becomes smaller, pulling up and opening out your cervix below. These are likely to be uncomfortable at first, growing steadily more painful as the contractions grow stronger.

The reduction of the womb and pulling up of your cervix creates the birth canal – a single passage of womb, opened cervix and vagina, down which your baby can pass to be born. At the end of this process is a brief stage called the transition, which some doctors recognize as a separate stage in itself.

The second stage, sometimes called the pushing stage of labour (because this is what you are doing), is divided into three parts. During the first, the baby is coming out of the bony cradle of your pelvis, and around at an angle into your vagina, described by the NCT as being like putting your foot into a Wellington boot. Your womb continues to contract powerfully, each one helping your baby to move another small part of the way along. During the third part, your baby is pushed out into the world. The whole of the second stage usually lasts 30 to 60 minutes, but it can take as little as a few minutes or be as long as two or more hours.

The third stage is when your womb expels the placenta out through your vagina. This takes anything from a few minutes, if you have been given an injection to speed the process up, to half an hour or more if no stimulants are used.

THE ONSET OF LABOUR

People tend to treat a heavily pregnant woman with immense caution, as if she is an unexploded bomb – likely to detonate at any minute. But general lifting (perhaps of a toddler or bags of shopping) walking extensively, sexual intercourse, even bumps and minor falls are unlikely to cause labour to start if it is not ready to do so. Labour is probably set in motion by the baby itself, with hormonal secretions from its own endocrine glands, which cross the placenta into the mother's bloodstream and stimulate her endocrine system to produce hormones which make her uterus begin contracting.

Your labour could begin in many different ways, but in general early signs include:

1. Regular contractions of the womb which come and go, and which become painful after a while.

2. The loss of some blood-stained discharge from your vagina. This is the plug of mucus which has been sealing off the cervix, protecting the unborn baby above. It is dislodged when the neck of the womb starts being taken up (see p. 24). This is called the show.

3. Your waters may break. This does not hurt, but some women report feeling a distinct pop or ping sensation. What has happened is that the membranes forming the amniotic sac, which keeps the baby surrounded in warm fluid, have ruptured. This is not always an indication your labour has started.

Any of the above can indicate that labour has begun, but none guarantee that it has definitely done so. It is sometimes difficult to tell for sure, and the following things may confuse matters:

● Strong and regular Braxton-Hicks contractions (see p. 19) in the last part of your pregnancy can be mistaken for first stage contractions.

● Women having their second, third (or subsequent) baby, tend to find that their body moves into labour more smoothly than it did for the first child.

● If it is your first baby, you may not be sure whether the process has begun because you have not felt labour contractions before and have nothing to compare with what you are feeling now.

FALSE LABOUR

Sometimes women have false labours, when their contractions seem to begin, but then fade away again without becoming stronger and more frequent.

This can happen at intervals for a couple of weeks before you really do go into labour. They may be caused by your womb contracting as it slowly manoeuvres your baby's head into the right position deep in the lower part of your pelvis.

These false labour contractions are usually a prelude to real labour and, frustrating though they can be, at least they tell you that your baby's birth is very near indeed.

I kept getting false labour pains for 12 days. They felt pretty strong to me, and every time I got really excited. The first few times, I immediately phoned my friends, my husband, my mother, the hospital. It was my first baby and I was all keyed up. Then each time – nothing. Then my family and friends started phoning me back asking – has it happened yet? And, meaning to be funny, 'Haven't you had it by now?' It got so I'd burst into tears every time they asked me and I had never felt such a failure in my whole life. So my husband bought a cheap answerphone and recorded one word on it: 'No.'

If you are having your baby at home, ring and report any of the above (or anything else unusual) to your midwife. If you are having your baby in hospital, phone the labour ward and talk to the midwife on duty. She will either advise you to come in to hospital, or to stay at home for a few hours more, depending on the symptoms you describe to her.

WHAT IS HAPPENING WHEN I HAVE CONTRACTIONS?

The muscles of your womb are working. Womb muscles are structured differently to other muscle masses. They are laid down in a series of spirals of about two turns each, which form a mirror image of each other, so that pulling on the left-hand spiral combined with a similar pull on its right-hand counterpart reduces the size of the womb. Unlike other muscles in your body, the muscle fibres of the womb become slightly shorter and fatter each time they clench or contract. Because the muscles do not revert to their former size after they have finished contracting, the womb gradually becomes smaller.

The overall effect of womb contractions is that they:

- tighten and reduce the size of the uterus, so it becomes gradually smaller
- pull up on, and dilate, the cervix until it has flattened out and become wide open
- push the baby deeper down into the pelvis.

The pattern of contractions varies. To start with they may last 10 seconds and arrive 30 to 45 minutes apart at the beginning of your labour, building up to 60-second contractions only one or two minutes apart just before you give birth. Alternatively you may find that your labour begins with not-very-strong contractions about three minutes apart, which will stay at roughly this frequency but become slowly more and more powerful.

People often wonder at what point they should call their midwife or go to hospital. If in any doubt at all, telephone for advice. In general, you'll be in plenty of time to wait until contractions are about 15 minutes apart. Usually it takes time to give birth, so there is no need to go straight to hospital as soon as any irregular pains begin.

In early labour (provided your waters have not broken) you may want to carry on with ordinary gentle activities like going for a walk, cooking, playing with any children you may have already, tidying up, relaxing in a warm bath (this should not be too hot, as it could also raise the baby's temperature). Some women find they want to start cleaning vigorously – the stories of women in labour feeling a strong desire to scrub kitchen floors are real.

If you have been taught relaxation, Autogenic Training, breathing, or self-hypnosis, now is a very good time to start practising some of what you have been learning if you have some peace and quiet so that you can stay as loose and relaxed as possible between contractions. This will help to prevent muscular tension building up in areas like your neck and shoulders. If your partner can help you with this, or do some massage for you, so much the better.

If your contractions become:
- regular
- much closer together
- the pain begins in the small of your back and radiates right around to the front just above your pubic bone

it is time to contact your hospital or midwife.

If you have had a baby before, you will probably give birth to subsequent babies faster. If you are going into hospital do so when your contractions are coming every 20 to 25 minutes rather than every 15 to be sure of getting there in time to make the best use of the facilities on offer including certain types of pain relief.

HOW TO TELL THE DIFFERENCE BETWEEN A BRAXTON-HICKS CONTRACTION AND A FIRST-STAGE CONTRACTION

Most women notice their womb hardening at intervals during pregnancy, especially if you put your hand on your abdomen wall. These are limbering up, practice contractions. While these are usually a sensation rather than feeling uncomfortable, they may be strong enough to make you catch your breath or stop still for a moment. You can also have less strong ones through which you can continue talking to someone or walking along.

If you are in labour, the contractions tend to produce a more definite discomfort or pain. Early on, they feel like:

i)　Period pains (anything from mild, familiar twinges to a swiping, slicing pain across the lower abdomen)

ii)　A low, sick, heavy backache

iii)　Abdominal cramps: many women say they thought they just had indigestion when they were in early labour

iv)　Pains down the inside of the thighs, in the hips, or even in the knees

v)　Pain and discomfort in the rectum which feels like constipation

Labour contractions	*Braxton Hicks contractions*
Become stronger and closer together as the hours pass, forming a pattern (eg every 45, 30 or 10 minutes)	Do not become closer together; remain irregular, showing no pattern
Build up into a peak of intensity each time, then die away again	Stay the same

Just how painful (or not) these contractions are depends on the woman experiencing them: how relaxed she is, how physically comfortable, what position she is sitting, standing, or lying in, and on her own physiological level of pain perception. Contraction intensity can be measured mechanically, using sensors attached to your abdomen wall. These are usually left on for about half an hour to get a recording of your contraction pattern when you first go into hospital in labour, and possibly at intervals after that. You usually register pain when the pressure rises to about 20mm on the register and lasts for 50 seconds or so. The contractions however go on for two or three minutes in all, with the beginning and end not feeling painful. Later in labour the pressure of a contraction can rise up to over 100mm and feel even more painful.

These traces do not always reflect accurately the amount of pain

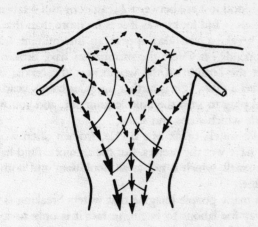

This diagram shows the way in which electrical pain impulses
begin at the top of the womb and flow down through it during
the next 15 to 20 seconds.

you are feeling – a 90mm peak score can be far more painful later
in labour when the muscles are tired, short of blood and building
up acidic waste products inside (see pp. 44–5).

It is thought that the womb's contractions begin from a pair
of pacemakers in the upper part of the womb, just where the
Fallopian tubes join it. They cause a regular wave of electrical
impulses to flow through the muscle fibre of the womb (see fig.
1), spreading right down its length.

As labour continues, with each contraction the womb axis tilts
slightly forward to encourage the baby's head into the right position so it can enter the birth canal.

WHAT IS HAPPENING WHEN MY WATERS BREAK?

This may feel like a gush of fluid, though it is usually only between
2–4 tablespoons and a cupful, because liquid coming from the
vagina always feels like more than it actually is. It is the same

when you bleed during a period – while the actual amounts of menstrual blood lost are between 2 teaspoons and 4 tablespoons, it always feels – and looks – as if it is far more than that.

Waters breaking can also appear an intermittent trickle. It entirely depends on where the membranes have broken. If the break is at the bottom of the womb near the cervix, you will probably feel a gush. If it is further up, your baby's head will act as a partial plug to stop the fluid leaking out, and you will only feel a trickle which stops and starts.

When the waters break as a trickle, women often worry that they must have wet themselves, but the amniotic fluid has a very distinctive smell, which is not at all unpleasant and nothing like that of urine.

Though many people imagine that waters breaking is the traditional way for labour to begin, in fact it is only so for about 10 per cent of women, being more common for mothers who have had babies before and less so for first-time mothers.

Your waters can break as much as a day or so before labour actually begins (this happens for about 4 per cent of all women). For a very small number of women it may even be several weeks before, in which case they would have to be admitted to hospital to help prevent a premature labour.

As to the most usual time of day – there isn't one. People often say that the commonest time for it to happen is when you are in bed, but this is probably because you will be there for about 8 hours in every 24, the longest time you are likely to be staying in one place in a 24-hour period.

Many women are concerned that their waters will break somewhere public and potentially embarrassing, but in fact they are no more likely to do so when you are out and about than at any other time. If you are concerned about this you can always wear a highly absorbent continence pad (like a larger sanitary towel, but still discreet) when you go out during your Due Week. These are available from any major chemist. For the same reason, and because the quantity of fluid lost can vary, many women also buy a rubber undersheet, placed beneath the bottom sheet halfway down the bed to protect the mattress from becoming wet. Or you can cut open a large binliner and use that as a mattress protector instead.

If you do lose what appears to be a good deal of fluid when your membranes break, do not worry that you will have what some people call a dry labour. More fluid is being made by the lining of the womb all the time, so the amount you will have inside you after another few hours will not be affected by what came out earlier.

The breaking of your waters can also intensify and speed up labour, sometimes quite dramatically, because the baby's head can press more directly against your cervix if it is no longer cushioned by a sac of amniotic fluid. This leads to an increase in the supply of oxytocin, the hormone which causes your womb to contract. Some obstetricians also suggest that the sac membranes themselves contain a hormone which encourages the womb to contract and that this too is released when they rupture.

STEP BY STEP – THE STAGES OF LABOUR

THE FIRST STAGE

This is the stage when the birth canal is prepared for the baby to pass down it.

Throughout pregnancy the cervix at the bottom or neck of the womb has been holding in the increasing weight of the baby and its surrounding membranes. As the baby has grown, the pressure on the cervix has increased – but in most women it has faithfully remained closed. For the very few women whose cervix does begin to open too early under the pressure, a cervical stitch can help a little to prevent premature labour.

In just the few hours of labour the neck of the womb has to transform itself from the baby's guardian, holding him or her in place, to a wide open, smooth tunnel for the baby to move down. This is a complete change in function and it has to make this change fast by stretching within a matter of hours from closed or almost closed to 10cm wide (see fig. 2).

This is one of the reasons why contractions in labour hurt, whilst

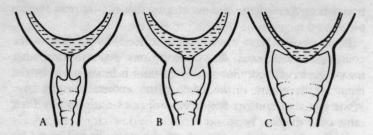

During labour the cervix pulls up, flattens out (effaces) then begins
to dilate (open up), eventually leaving a gap measuring about 10cm
across through which the baby can be born. In (a) the cervix is
shown in pregnancy before it has changed shape at all; (b) shows
it beginning to be taken up; and (c) shows it taken up and
beginning to dilate – here it has reached about 2cm across and the
baby's head, in its sac of amniotic fluid, is pushing down against it.

those earlier in pregnancy tend not to. During pregnancy there may
have been some passive cervical dilation due to the pressure of the
baby and its surrounding fluid – which is why some women are
already 1–2cm dilated even before they go into labour.

When the uterus pulls on the cervix to open it up, it is like
taking a sock with a small hole in the tip and pulling it up over
your foot – then continuing to pull gently. Your big toe would
make the hole in that sock slightly bigger each time you pulled
it. And if you went on pulling intermittently, eventually the hole
would become big enough for the other toes to come out through
there too, and eventually, your entire foot. Something very similar
happens to your cervix when you are in labour – except it closes
up again neatly afterwards.

Most women find labour painful to some extent, though
according to the Russian obstetrician Velvoski up to 10 per cent
of Russian mothers say they are only conscious of major physical
effort and 'something happening'. Any pain in labour comes not
directly from your womb itself, but from ischaemia – a lack of
blood in the abdominal tissues caused by the womb squeezing
and contracting.

This hurts for the same reason as a heart attack or angina pain hurts: lack of oxygen to the muscles and a build-up of cell waste products which can be irritating to nerve tissue.

Some women like to move about as freely as possible in the first stage: to walk, squat, lean over cushions, chairs and beanbags, float in water and get into several different positions in or out of the water, depending on what feels most comfortable at the time. Some prefer to remain upright or mobile as the pain increases, others find they get tired and prefer to lie down for a rest, ideally on their side to ensure maximum blood supply to the baby.

If you feel you would like some pharmacological pain relief, now is the time to ask for it. Many methods, especially the stronger ones like epidurals, need time to take effect. Even pethidine takes time; most people think of it as immediately available, for it can be given by your midwife rather than waiting for a doctor, but it has first to be fetched from the drug cupboard and, because it is a scheduled drug, the midwife will need another midwife to co-sign for it before injecting it into your muscle. After that, it takes another 20 minutes to work, which in all adds up to at least 30–50 minutes from the time you first asked for it.

Though the contractions cause your cervix to dilate, this is not an even process; it can progress from tightly shut to wide open in fits and starts. Dilation is also a highly individual process, like the rest of childbirth. One woman may go very slowly from 2cm to 5cm, then suddenly progress very swiftly to 10cm. Another may go quickly to 4 or 5cm then appear to stop there for a while, before moving on.

If you are having a second or subsequent baby, you may find that your cervix dilates very fast, especially after you have got about halfway there.

By the end of the first stage your baby's head has nudged right down into the cavity within your pelvis, but there may be a small amount of cervix left which has yet to dilate out of the way, or has done so unevenly, leaving a small area behind. This is called a lip. If you get an urge to push the baby out when this lip is in place, it will become swollen and make it difficult to finish dilating.

To stop yourself from pushing at this point, it can help if you get into a position where you are on all fours with your forehead touching the ground and your bottom up in the air. Alternatively, breathing nitrous oxide and oxygen can give some pain relief, and may stop the urge to push too soon.

Eating and drinking

Many hospitals have not, in the past, been keen to let women in labour eat anything. This is probably because of the very slight possibility that if there are any major problems and you need an emergency caesarean under general anaesthetic, you might vomit up anything that was in your stomach at the time. When someone vomits under general anaesthetic there is a risk of inhaling the stomach's contents into the lungs, which would flood with fluid as a result. But this can usually be avoided by careful management of the tube which is passed down an anaesthetized patient's throat during any operation.

Some primitive societies also forbid eating during labour. The Tiwi of Australia believe 'food slows the birth', the Jukun of Nigeria that it hinders childbirth. A few tribes even refuse women in labour sips of water. But most cultures see nothing wrong with a light snack, if the woman feels she wants it – and most labouring women do not eat much because they are too busy concentrating on other things.

Labour is a huge physical effort and you may find you would welcome something light to eat at intervals to keep your energy level up. Some of the American Indian peoples offer warm soups, a Lepcha mother would be given a little meat from a fowl or goat, and if it looks as if a Vietnamese mother is tiring she would be offered a bowl of rice with an egg.

Convenient and helpful foods for British women could be anything light that was made partially of complex carbohydrates, as they release their energy slowly and steadily into the system. There is no good reason why a woman in labour cannot eat these if she wants to, preferably a bit at a time – as long as she avoids a major meal or anything that is especially difficult to digest, such as salad. Try:

A banana

A few digestive biscuits

Wholemeal sandwiches of honey, peanut butter – or any other favourite filling

Chicken soup

But let your midwife know that you have had something to eat.

As for drinking, plain water is best. Sweet fizzy drinks are not a good idea because they slow down the absorption of fluids from your gut.

TRANSITION

Many obstetricians deny that this counts as a separate stage of labour in its own right, but those who say it is explain it as the time when the womb changes the way it is contracting, from spasms which reduce the womb in size and dilate the cervix to those which can powerfully push the baby out into the world. You may not notice transition at all. But you may have one or more of the following symptoms:

- You may feel sick
- You may have diarrhoea
- You may shake uncontrollably, or feel very cold
- You may find your contractions no longer seem to have a pattern to them, or that it is no longer possible to cope with them
- You might find you are either confused mentally or extremely irritable and upset. This is often the point at which a mother may suddenly become very angry with her partner, possibly shouting at them, ordering them to go away, or blaming them for the pain she is having. Some women say they felt they no longer wanted to have their baby at all, or that they had suddenly had enough and wanted it all to be over immediately. Others mention that they just wanted to go home – now – or found it difficult if not impossible to co-operate with those around them

- You may not want to be touched, helped or comforted – merely to be left alone by everyone
- You may have a premature urge to begin pushing, possibly as a result of the baby's head pressing hard on your rectum
- You may start to feel there is light at the end of the tunnel and the end of labour is approaching.

THE SECOND STAGE

This is the time when your baby is born. It starts when the cervix is fully dilated to 10cm. At its narrowest diameter your baby's head is also about 10cm, provided it is in the best position (see pp. 30–5 below). So it is not too big to be slowly and steadily pushed through the opened cervix, as if through the polo neck of a jumper.

From being fully dilated to giving birth to your baby can take a few swift contractions, or up to three hours. The usual time is between 30 and 60 minutes.

As you go into the second stage, your contractions will probably feel about the same all the way through, instead of building up to a climax.

You may also feel:

- as if you have suddenly got an extra burst of energy;
- excited ('This is it at last . . .');
- a strong, often irresistible urge to push or bear down. Do not worry if you are not able to co-ordinate your pushing very well, as it is the womb which is still automatically doing most of the work. Women often manage to deliver their babies without extra help even when they have had an epidural and have little or no sensation in the lower part of their body;
- as if you want to open your bowels. This is because of the strong pressure of your baby's head against your rectum. But the rectum is usually empty anyway (faeces tend to be

stored a few inches further up in the colon), so it is not a sensation from inside your bowel caused by waste matter but one from the outside. Your neurological system, however, is being thoroughly overloaded in this area so it cannot tell the difference. Do not worry if you do move your bowels slightly – this is quite usual and it is going to be no surprise to midwives or doctors. They will take no notice of it at all, apart from just removing any faecal matter swiftly with a piece of gauze and throwing it away.

Boosting

Women in labour may also become tired or discouraged at this point and it is now they need all the encouragement and praise that their partner or midwife can give them.

Now that it can pass its head through your cervix, the baby has to manoeuvre its way through the rest of the birth canal. This is not a straight tube but a curved one rather like the U-bend at the bottom of a drainpipe. Nor is it equally wide all the way through. At the top, it is widest from side to side, and at the outlet (the exit of the vagina) it is widest from front to back. This means that the baby's head has to rotate and turn as it comes down the birth canal, and so must its shoulders which will follow later.

This happens naturally as the baby's descent follows the muscle and bony walls of the pelvis, but it can take a little while. At the beginning of the second stage the baby's head is usually in the traverse position, following the lines of your pelvis as it descends (figs. 3 and 4).

When your baby first comes into contact with the air, the change in temperature makes it automatically take a breath and fill its lungs. It may take a little time before it is breathing efficiently.

If the baby's breathing is inhibited by mucus in its nose or throat the staff will check and clear this. Should the baby need additional help, hospitals have all the necessary resuscitation equipment, plus the appropriate antidotes for conditions caused by pain-relieving drugs like pethidine which can sometimes interfere with a newborn baby's breathing mechanisms (see p. 108).

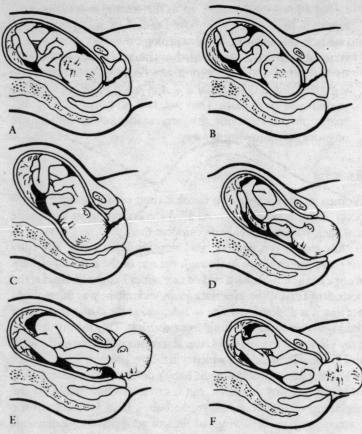

A

B

C

D

E

F

(A) At first, the baby's head needs to be flexed so the chin is resting against the chest. This means the smallest possible diameter of the head (about 10cm) is leading the rest of the body down into the mother's pelvis. If, however, the head is not well flexed, the leading part will measure nearer 13cm across, and this can make things much more difficult.

(B) As baby's head reaches the mother's pelvic floor it rotates about 90 degrees to face the base of the mother's spine.

(C) The head then passes under the pubic bone and into the top of the vagina.

(D) Now the back of the baby's head extends from the neck – like a diver coming up for air in slow motion – and, after a little more descent, the head is born.

(E) The baby rotates sideways as its shoulders are now entering the mother's pelvis and they need to follow the same graceful turning motion as the head did. This usually happens quite quickly, with the midwife holding the baby's head gently but firmly to support it.

(F) The baby now turns and faces mother's thigh, as its shoulders are delivered. The body bends first sideways towards the back so the uppermost shoulder is freed, then towards the front to free the other shoulder. The widest part is now out and the rest of the body follows smoothly and easily.

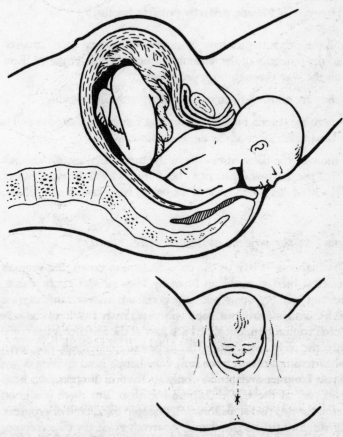

The baby's head having been born, the rest of the body will follow.

How does something as large as a baby manage to pass down the vagina?

Many women worry about this. While they know it is technically what happens – and what has happened for many thousands of years – the idea of something the size of a baby's head passing down a slim passageway like the vagina seems somehow beyond all reason.

However it *is* made perfectly possible because:

- all the pelvic tissues have by now become very elastic, thanks to the influence of the relaxing hormone progesterone on them all the way through your pregnancy;

- they are allowed to stretch slowly, gently and steadily;

- there are several birth positions that can encourage your pelvis to naturally open up as far as possible;

- the way the baby comes down the birth canal usually ensures that the narrowest part of its head always leads the way. Where the head can go, the rest of the baby's body can usually follow.

How can the vagina stretch so well?

What happens is that as the baby is coming down, the vagina's surface, which is made up of many folds of soft elastic tissue, stretches steadily apart and the perineum tissues fan out (see fig. 5). This means your baby will pass down a little of the way at each contraction, but slide back part of the distance it has come when the contraction stops. It can be extremely frustrating, even disheartening, to watch (or feel) your baby's head coming down as you contract and push – only to have it disappear back up again part of the way each time you stop. But there is a good reason for this two steps forward, one step back, type of progress. It gives your tissues the chance to stretch gradually to accommodate the baby moving down, and thus reduces the risk of them tearing.

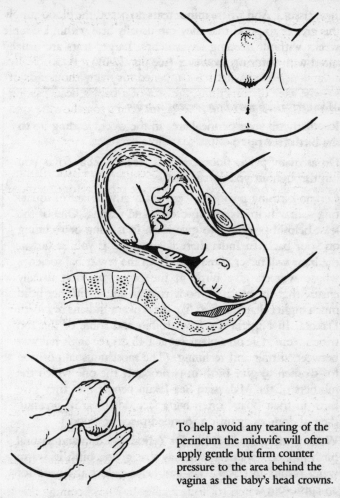

To help avoid any tearing of the perineum the midwife will often apply gentle but firm counter pressure to the area behind the vagina as the baby's head crowns.

Furthermore, because of the large quantities of hormones that have been circulating in your system throughout pregnancy and labour, all the tissues and ligaments in your entire pelvic area are exceptionally soft and stretchy. So when you give birth, your baby is usually able squeeze out with little or no trouble.

About one in three women do not have even the smallest tear

in these tissues. And where minor tears do occur, the blood supply to this area is so good that they can usually heal within a couple of weeks without needing any stitches. Larger tears are usually repaired with suturing, however (see pp. 274ff).

Measures which may help prevent tearing

Regularly oil your perineal area in the weeks leading up to the birth (see pp. 6–7).

Do as many pelvic floor exercises (see pp. 285–9) as you can throughout your pregnancy.

Certain birthing positions – especially any variant of squatting – may help avoid episiotomy and tearing. One of the least helpful positions to give birth in is lying or reclining on your back. In India there is a saying: 'If you lie down, the baby will never come out.' Even the few tribal societies whose women give birth in the prone position usually ensure that the mother's body is at an angle with her head much higher than her feet, like the Arikara Indians of North Dakota. In Nigeria the Ijaw, Ibibio and some of the Ibo tribe's women lie on a plank set at a 45 degree angle halfway between sitting and reclining. (The most unusual position for women to give birth in is probably the one which the mothers of the Malaysian Sea-Jakun people use: they give birth in their boats, often lying face downwards, pressing their abdomens against a rounded piece of wood.)

Water birth enthusiasts like Dr Yehudi Gordon and natural birth pioneer Janet Balaskas say that giving birth in warm water results in fewer tears and helps reduce the need for an episiotomy.

The midwife should protect the perineum with gentle but firm counterpressure as the baby's head crowns.

Holding comfortingly hot compresses against the perineal area during the second stage of labour can also help the tissues relax and stretch more (see p. 7).

THE THIRD STAGE

This is when the placenta is squeezed off its attachment to the wall of the womb, and delivered through the vagina.

As the womb contracts and shrinks, the placenta attached to it crumples up and peels away, rather like a large sticky label peeling away from a rapidly deflating balloon. This exposes the mother's blood vessels which have been supplying the placenta with blood throughout pregnancy, but they close down rapidly as the womb continues shrinking. The placenta passes down into the lower part of the womb and is expelled, along with the membranes and some clots of blood, by the next few contractions.

The midwife may help this process along by giving an injection of artificial oxytocic to stimulate uterine contractions. This can ensure that the placenta is delivered within minutes rather than the half hour or so it would take to do so naturally; but it is more often done to prevent heavy bleeding than for the mother's comfort. The midwife might also apply very gentle traction on the umbilical cord to which the placenta is attached. On no account should she pull it hard, as this itself can cause a haemorrhage.

It takes a few weeks for the womb to get back to its usual dimensions. By then, it will have shrunk from the size and shape of a very large melon or pumpkin to nearer that of a very small pear.

During this period, the place where the placenta was attached to the uterus wall will continue to bleed a little until it heals. This blood loss is called lochia, and you may notice it more if you are breastfeeding because the baby's suckling stimulates the release of oxytocic, which causes your womb to contract. These contractions may be felt as afterpains, which can range from the barely noticeable to 'as bad as labour pains themselves' (see pp. 220–22 for advice on how to soothe these).

What Does It Feel Like?

Labour pain may feel reassuringly familiar – many women describe the pain in the first stage of labour as being similar to their period pains, only stronger.

In 1994 100 mothers at St George's Hospital, London, were asked to describe what labour felt like. Here are some of their comments on the first stage:

'Not painful – I just felt like my stomach was heaving and I needed to throw up'

'A dull ache in my lower back'

'Stabbing pains'

'Slicing, sideswiping pains'

'A grinding, sickening, heavy ache in my back/belly'

'Slicing pain across the top of my pubic hair area'

'Stabs of sharp pain going down my inside thighs'

'Like a fat cord being pulled increasingly tighter, then releasing around my middle'

'I just thought it was bad wind'

'It felt like I had eaten something bad – there were twisting pains in my guts that came and went'

'Like this huge hand squeezing my guts on and off'

LABOUR PAIN

The pains ranged in severity from 'excruciating' and 'no one told me it would be like this' to 'not half as bad as I expected' and 'I've never understood why people make such a big thing of it. The baby's the thing to make a fuss about'. For some the experience was simply 'exciting' or 'hard work – they don't call it "labour" for nothing – but not painful as such', or 'painful, but I could handle it somehow'.

One very important thing to know about labour pain is that it is made easier to cope with than other sorts of pain because, unlike the pain of, say, slamming your hand in a door, which will hurt severely and constantly, labour pain comes and goes.

Unless your labour is being artificially accelerated (see p. 76) the pain will start gently and then gradually increase in severity over the next 30–60 seconds to peak for perhaps 10 seconds, after which it starts to die away, finally stopping altogether. Then you get a rest from it for a while. At the beginning of labour you would have 15 or 20 minutes' rest before your next contraction began. Towards the end of the first stage contractions will probably be coming every couple of minutes, but you should still be getting invaluable breaks in between.

Early in labour you will be able to carry on talking or walking through a mild contraction. As labour progresses, the contractions will be strong enough to make you stop moving and want to bend over, lean against something, practise relaxation breathing, squat down, or get down on all fours until the pain passes. Nor will you be able to carry on talking through these later contractions, as you will probably find that they take your breath away. As the first stage of labour approaches its end you are likely to find that you have neither the inclination nor the energy to talk, except to communicate information very briefly – such as 'Rub harder' or 'Need a drink' or 'mask, now'.

Because labour pains are gradual, wave-like and intermittent, you will:

- Have enough notice to prepare yourself to cope as you feel one beginning (whether by practising breathing or relaxation, requesting extra back-rubbing, or reaching out for the Entonox mask)

- Know that when it is at its most intense it is not going to last long – perhaps 10 to 30 seconds – before it starts wearing off again

> • Have rest periods in which to recover, move about, relax and regain your strength in between each one.

The second stage, when you are pushing your baby down the birth canal and out into the world to be born, involves sensations from the strong pushing you are doing and also from the stretching of your vagina, perineum and labia.

> The women in our survey described giving birth as:
> 'Like trying to pass an enormous, hard bowel motion when very constipated'
>
> 'Like trying to pass a melon out'
>
> 'Like a Chinese burn' *(Describing the feeling when the birth canal tissues stretch wide as the baby passes)* 'A splitting, tearing feeling'
>
> 'A massive stretching, but no pain' *(This is often the case as the tissues are temporarily stretched far enough to obliterate any of the usual neurological pain messages from them)* 'I felt plenty as the baby was coming down but nothing apart from a slithering, sliding – like she was toothpaste being squeezed from a tube – after the main part of her head was through'
>
> 'Nothing. I had an epidural, which was a Godsend. I was trying to help push, but the midwife said that I need not bother as 80 per cent of the power came from automatic womb contracting and only 20 per cent would be my pushing deliberately, so the baby would come out anyway with or without help from me'

According to the 1990 NBT survey, the sewing up of any tears after birth can hurt almost as much as labour itself if the area is not properly anaesthetized. If it *is* properly anaesthetized, it should not hurt. It is therefore very important that anaesthetic be given enough time – from three to six minutes, on average – to work.

'The worst part was the stitching'

'No episiotomy implies minimum pain *subsequent* to delivery, which is just as significant as pain during delivery' *(a partner's view)*

'I felt that the stitches were worse than the whole labour stages one, two and three. Although I had gas and an injection they were still very painful'

'I could still feel them stitching and it really hurt, even after an injection. So they gave me another and that was OK. The doctor was very good. He was rushed off his feet but he waited until the second had taken effect before starting again'

'I could still feel it after two injections, but they told me I could not have any more'

'It had been a really good birth and I had coped with the pain fine. The stitching up afterwards spoilt it all'

You may need more than one shot of anaesthetic as the area is now very sensitive as well as torn, and possibly swollen too.

So if you can feel the stitching, insist they stop and give you some more pain relief there. If this has no effect, tell your partner to insist on your behalf.

WHY DOES CHILDBIRTH HURT SOME WOMEN LESS THAN OTHERS? AND WHY IS IT USUALLY QUICKER AND EASIER SECOND TIME AROUND?

The answers to these two questions are closely linked and involve a combination of several different factors, both physical and psychological. Bravery in the face of pain is not one of them.

'It would be futile and ignorant to criticize someone's inability to cope with pain or to call them a coward if they are finding it more difficult than others to manage,' says Dr Christopher Wells,

Director of the Pain Research Unit at the Walton Hospital, Liverpool. 'Pain is a sensory *and* an emotional experience for the sufferer. It is not directly related to tissue damage. It is related to distress.'

Dr Wells uses the analogy of a radio to explain pain and the reasons why people experience it differently:

> 'When you switch on a radio to, say, Radio 1, everyone will be receiving the same signal. However, the volume on some people's sets will be turned down low, on others it will be turned up higher. The signal remains the same. It is a question of how loud it is being played.
>
> The radio owner controls the volume, not the signal. It is the same with pain. The stimulus is the same for everyone, but they can turn the volume of it up or down with a variety of factors which either allow more pain signal through (fear, anxiety) or compete with the pain signals (analgesic drugs, water, massage, TENS, acupuncture, distraction therapy).
>
> This means that a woman who is feeling nervous or under-confident is not, as some might suggest, getting herself in a state and imaging she is in great pain – she *is* in great pain.'

WHAT INFLUENCES HOW LITTLE OR HOW MUCH PAIN YOU FEEL IN LABOUR?

1 *Whether you have had a baby before*: From a physical point of view, for the second or subsequent births your cervix will be less resistant to being dilated, and your vagina and perineum will stretch a little more easily. Some also say that the body seems to remember what to do, and it is certainly true that you are less likely to have problems with the birth getting started properly, or with apparently ineffective womb contractions. Also, you may know more about childbirth and understand it better – and therefore be more relaxed and confident with later babies than you were with your first. Relaxation and confidence can reduce pain.

'My first baby Ben took 17 hours and I had an accelerating drip, an epidural which was only partially effective and wore off after a couple of hours; and then no more pain relief – the lot. I would say, even looking back five years later, that it was terribly painful. Yet my second, Jessie, arrived in four hours (mostly in the last five minutes when I went from 3cm dilation to delivery like a rocket) and apart from those few minutes where I simply did not know what to do with myself except hang on in there, it was perfectly manageable.'

'Sian took 15 hours to arrive. For three years afterwards I couldn't face the idea of even trying to get pregnant again. But the second time, I remember thinking: 'Here we go again – let's get on with it' and four hours later, Zoe was out and yelling her head off. It was very strange but it was as if I sort of remembered what I needed to do at each bit as it came along.'

'My second and third babies' labours felt almost familiar – and exciting. The less said about the first, the better.'

'I didn't believe what my friends kept telling me – that the second one is much easier. I thought they were just trying to make me feel better. But its true. Now other mums pregnant with their second do not believe me when I try and tell *them*.'

2 *Your age*: Research has shown that labour can be less painful for younger women.

3 *Social influences and family background*: What your own mother and friends say about their experiences of labour – if they discuss it at all – can greatly influence your expectations.

4 *Your periods*: If you have mild periods, you may be more likely to have an easier time in labour.

5 *Culture*: Winifred Francis, emeritus consultant obstetrician at the Liverpool Maternity Hospital, compared the way Nordic and Slav women experienced childbirth with the way Italian women felt, and found a vast difference. In Italy it is widely accepted that someone in pain should feel free to make as much noise as they need to, as a way of coping with it. But women from Nordic countries seem to approach labour in a far more controlled way, often saying little even though they are in great pain and might be helped by pain relief. 'It takes a good midwife to recognize these differences and be able to help accordingly,' says Dr Christopher Wells.

6 *How much you understand about what is happening to you*: Women are far better informed about childbirth now than they were 30 years ago, thanks to more frequent (and welcoming) hospital antenatal/parentcraft classes, the work of NCT and Active Childbirth organizations, and the availability of a host of books and magazines about pregnancy, birth and babies.

The effect of mothers understanding more about labour may be one reason for the sharp drop in the average time spent in labour since the early 1960s. The average labour time for a first-time mother has come down from ten hours to seven, while the average time for subsequent labours has dropped from nine hours to four.

7 *Confidence in your own ability to manage*: Factors 1, 3 and 6 all play a part in boosting your confidence. This is one of the reasons it's so much easier second time around.

8 *An ability to relax*: Again, 1, 3, 6 and 7 above all play a part in determining how much you are able to relax while in labour.

9 *Whether your labour is being artificially accelerated*: If it is, it is likely to be more painful as contractions will probably be sharper and much closer together (see p. 76).

WHY LABOUR HURTS AT ALL

PHYSICAL REASONS FOR LABOUR PAINS

Why do animals – and other primates, who are physically similar to humans – seem to give birth so easily and most humans find it harder? One reason is an evolutionary imperfection in human beings: we are the only primates whose babies' heads are larger than the entrance to the birth canal.

Scientists believe this came about because, in order to be able to stand upright and become a hunter-gatherer rather than a fruit-eating tree inhabitant, the human ape's pelvis needed to become narrower than that of an ordinary ape, and to change from a cylinder shape with a round cross section to a curve with a more irregular cross section. (If you are ever in a natural history museum and come across a skeleton of a gorilla or orang-utan, try bending down to look up its pelvis and you will see that cylinder shape, which makes a much simpler channel for a baby to be born through.)

However, while the human ape's pelvis was shrinking, its skull was expanding in order to accommodate its rapidly evolving brain. What with mothers' smaller pelvic girdles and babies' larger heads, the human infant's birth entrance into the world became something of a tight fit.

- The problem of the ratio of the baby's head to the mother's pelvis is exaggerated if the baby has a particularly large head, or if it is an especially big baby (which can happen when the mother is a diabetic) or when the mother has an especially small pelvic cavity.

- Contractions in the uterus: pain begins in the muscles of the uterus and peaks at the height of a contraction as the nerve fibres are stimulated by the squeezing of the muscles they are threaded through.

- The position of the baby (see pp. 30–35).

- Stretching in the cervix: pain comes from the stretching and dilating of the cervix as it opens up, and from the lower part of the uterus during contractions.

- Stretching in the ligaments of the pelvis, soft tissues and joints stimulates the nerves running through them.

- A reduction to the free flow of blood in and out of the muscles of the womb.

  Arterial blood delivers food, which is converted to energy, and oxygen; deoxygenated blood flows out, removing waste products. Interruptions to the flow can occur during labour because as muscles contract they squeeze and compress the blood vessels running through them, partially cutting off both the arterial supply of oxygenated blood to that area and the venous drainage routes leading away from it. The muscle area then becomes ischaemic or oxygen-starved. When a muscle is ischaemic it goes into spasm and this can be painful; the sharp pain of angina in the heart is due to this. No one is quite sure why this should hurt as it does, but one theory suggests it follows the progressive build-up of large amounts of cell waste products such as lactic acid, and that these can irritate the nerve endings.

- Muscle contraction also increases the rate of metabolism in all the tissues in the surrounding area. This can speed up the onset of pain.

- Tension builds up in muscles during labour and this makes them sore. Many women automatically find they stiffen and hunch their shoulders at the height of a major contraction, developing rigid, painful stiff shoulder and back muscles as a result. When muscles become stiff or tired they are far more vulnerable to injury such as tears and strains.

- In the second stage of labour, pain is also caused by the stretching of tissues in the vagina, vulva, perineum and the pushing further apart of the pelvic joints as the baby comes down the birth canal.

- The way in which different people react to different painkilling drugs: painkillers (analgesics) may have more of an effect on one woman than another. If it still hurts, it may be because your system is resistant to the action of the particular drug being used. Take no notice if the staff tell you 'Don't be silly, it can't possibly still be hurting', and keep complaining. Or better still, before you are in labour, sort out with your partner what they will do on your behalf should this happen (eg be insistent, or ask to see an anaesthetist).

PSYCHOLOGICAL REASONS

If you need a higher dose of painkiller than the next person because something is still hurting, it does not mean you are less brave than they are, or that you have a lower pain threshold than most. In fact, there are tests which can measure an individual's pain threshold – and the results show that it is about the same for everyone, as Dr Wells explains:

The Walton Pain Unit has done many experiments in which we ask someone to hold a metal rod in a laboratory and it is then slowly heated or frozen until they feel discomfort. Almost everybody's discomfort (pain) point is the same – 43°C for heat and -6°C for cold. What does vary from person to person is pain *tolerance* (the ability to cope with pain). And the amount of pain you can tolerate depends on your personal approach to it and a host of psychological factors.

These factors include:

Whether you are relaxed, or nervous: The less tense or anxious you are the less something is likely to hurt. There are good physiological reasons why fear makes pain worse and relaxation can reduce it. And they explain why so many of the non-drug methods of pain relief for labour are aimed at encouraging women to be calm and relaxed.

WHY ANXIETY = PAIN IN LABOUR

If a woman is calm and relaxed during childbirth this can substantially reduce any labour pain. However, if she becomes distressed or frightened when she is in labour, the amount of tension in her muscles increases and the level of natural opiates (endorphins) which the central nervous system usually secretes to soothe pain decreases. This will probably cause a longer labour and the mother will register more pain, which in turn may increase her anxiety still further – with the result that she will produce even smaller amounts of endorphins.

If her output of endorphins drops, a different group of hormones starts to be secreted instead. These are adrenaline-like substances called catecholamines, which would normally be released in the second stage of labour to stimulate the powerful, expulsive contractions of the womb. If catecholamines are secreted too soon, during the first stage, they can inhibit the contractions responsible for reducing the size of the womb and pulling up the cervix (see pp. 25–6). This is thought to increase the amount of pain felt by the mother. Moreover, catecholamines are pain transmitters in themselves, so the more of these there are around the more pain will be felt.

And so you get a vicious circle of anxiety/physical tension/increased perception of pain which can be very hard to break .

There are, however, many things that both the mother herself, her doctor, her midwife and her partner can do to help deal with any fear and nervousness she feels and encourage her to feel more relaxed. Some of the techniques, such as Autogenic Training and hypnosis, require practice beforehand. But many other techniques, including massage, warm water baths and showers, being read to, gentle music, aromatherapy oils, or homeopathic remedies can have a surprisingly calming effect and require no earlier practice, though for the latter two you do need to have taken the advice of a professional aromatherapist or homeopathist as to what to bring with you. A wide range of relaxation techniques is described in the chapter on **Non-Pharmacological Pain Relief**).

Whether you are expecting something to hurt: The very *expectation* of pain can hurt. When medical student volunteers at the Walton Pain Unit were told they were about to be subjected to terribly high temperatures which, if they did not press the 'cut-off button' in time, could cause severe tissue damage, they grimaced with pain and dropped the temperature rods they were holding. In fact, the machines were not even switched on at the time.

A memory of a previous childbirth can have the same effect. If it was a good experience you are likely to be expecting another. If the last birth was difficult and painful, you might fear a repeat and be more aware of the pain as a result. Being told very alarming stories by friends or relatives about painful labours they've had can have the same effect.

This may be one of the reasons why many doctors and midwives tend to play down the pain of childbirth – for fear of negatively prejudicing the outcome, on the grounds that if you tell someone it is going to hurt a lot, then it will. However, though they may mean well, they are misguided.

Just telling a pregnant woman that labour is pretty painful can be giving her an incomplete picture and is therefore not helpful.

It is not the same as telling her the truth – which is that her childbirth might hurt a lot or it might not, but if it does there is a great deal that can be done both by her, her partner, and the midwives and doctors to relieve this and/or help her cope with it.

Whether there is anything to distract you from the pain: Pain stimuli have to reach and register in the brain before you can feel them. If they are prevented from getting there, you won't be conscious of any hurt. If some are prevented from getting through you will be conscious of a degree of hurt. If they all get through you will feel a good deal of pain.

Though everyone has the same pain threshold, we have different levels of interruption along the route which pain signals travel to the brain. Other sensory stimuli can compete with pain signals and prevent many reaching the cerebral cortex where they register as discomfort. Treatments such as TENS, acupuncture, massage, water immersion, showers and distraction therapy all work in this way.

Whether you know there is a reward at the end of the pain: If pain has a good reason or you know that there will be a reward at the end of it, it makes it easier to cope with. When a group of student volunteers at the Centre for Pain Relief were told they would be paid well to take part in tests on pain sensitivity they were able to withstand far higher levels of pain stimulus than those who thought their efforts were purely in the interests of science with no payment involved.

'Women often say that their childbirth was indeed very painful at times but they could handle it because there was a joyful point to it all: their baby being born at the end,' says Dr Christopher Wells. 'Yet those whose baby died while in labour and who were told they were going to have a stillbirth found their labours far more painful than women who knew that they were going to have a live birth. I think this is because the reward of having their child at the end has been taken away from them.'

COUVADE

'There are more things in heaven and earth, Horatio, than are dreamt of in Eden & Holland's *Manual of Obstetrics*,' he told me darkly. 'Whenever Molly goes into labour, I get the most shocking bellyache.'

Dr Richard Gordon, *Doctor & Son*, 1959

Couvade (which means 'hatching pains' in French) describes the phenomenon whereby some men share their partner's childbirth pain.

There are well documented examples of this all over the world. Anthropologist Alan Merriam reports that when a woman of the Basongye tribe in Zaire goes into labour, the father 'apparently falls ill, complains of headache, stomach pains, loses his appetite, cannot even enjoy smoking. Men know the instant of the birth of their children because that is the instant their own symptoms disappear. Some people suggest that this may be due to worry about their wife and child, but numerous cases are also cited in which a man is far away from home, falls ill suddenly and recovers just as suddenly – then learns of his wife's delivery at these very moments.'

Arapesh fathers in New Guinea habitually writhe in pain when their wife is in labour; they are also the ones who receive all the congratulations and presents when the baby is born. In America, it used to be thought that if the woman crossed her husband's bed at the first sign of labour, he would then have to share in her pains.

But though couvade is widely recognized in tribal civilizations, most Western midwives and obstetricians (with a few notable exceptions, such as Michel Odent) say they see little evidence of it. So it is interesting that a small survey of 100 couples for this book carried out by the midwives of St George's Hospital revealed that, of the 49 men who replied, 3 had experienced severe backache or abdominal pain while their wife or girlfriend was in labour. More research is needed, but purely as a pilot study this suggests that couvade does still occur, and could affect up to 1 in 16 fathers.

WHY MIGHT MEN EXPERIENCE LABOUR PAINS?

Experts are so far unable to agree about why it can happen, but it may be that during childbirth the psychological ties between some men and women are stronger than anyone suspects. Theories range from the psychological to the supernatural:

- It is a mild form of clinical hysteria. If someone you are close to emotionally becomes exceptionally excited or agitated, you may find you get agitated too after a while in their company – literally, catching their mood.

- It is the father's way of showing sympathy for his wife during labour; he shares her suffering through a form of sympathetic magic. According to anthropologist Sir James George Frazer, author of *The Golden Bough*, sympathetic magic is the belief that you can make something happen by acting it out ritually yourself.

● Some psychoanalysts see couvade as a 'direct link with a man's wish to grow life within him' and suggest that it is associated with womb envy, the male equivalent of the penis envy women are supposed to experience.

● It is an instinctive way of trying to ward off any unfriendly supernatural forces. Many societies believe that there are harmful spirits which may be attracted to a woman in labour, both by the smell of blood and by her especial spiritual vulnerability at this time. Sometimes these forces are thought to be the sad spirits of women who themselves died in childbirth. The man therefore acts as a decoy, trying to take his wife's place to avert any spiritual dangers which may threaten her and the baby during, and soon after, its birth.

   Another traditional way of deceiving any loitering demons was for the woman to pretend to be her husband, getting up after giving birth and walking around for a while dressed in his hat and trousers.

   Alternatively, in the view of sociologist and philosopher Claude Levi Strauss, it is the baby who is considered most in need of protection and therefore the man is not playing out the wife's part but that of the child.

● According to French obstetrician Jacques Gelis it is, either consciously or unconsciously, a social rite the father performs in honour of the new baby, publicly recognizing and adopting the child as his.

● It occurs because the father feels the need to take an active part in the birth of his child.

In Ireland men in rural areas traditionally had such a role defined for them. When a woman went into labour her husband would often do some tiring (and symbolic) work like drawing water from a well. He would not stop until the baby was born, so matching his own major physical effort with his wife's. This type of ritual behaviour was thought to reduce some of the mother's pain by transferring it to the father.

Many modern fathers find they have nothing specific to do while their partners are in labour. They talk of feeling helpless, even irrelevant while their partner is going through childbirth. They say they felt as if they had no role to play at a time when something very important (which they helped begin) was coming to its climax. Some report that they wanted to have a proper place in the proceedings but could find none; instead they felt ignored or shut out because everyone's attention was totally focused on the mother.

So for some men, it may be that sharing the woman's pain is the one way they feel they can have a legitimate part to play in the birth process. It may also be that they are prepared to cause pain to themselves either as a mark of love, support and respect for their partner, or to help counterbalance their own feeling of powerlessness and temporarily not mattering.

Fathers' comments:

'I felt in the way, and worried about doing the wrong thing.'

'I was in tears because I felt so useless – she was in such pain and I could not help her.'

'It was my baby too and I wanted to do something, anything. So I rubbed her back. For hours, it felt like, till my shoulders ached. It helped Elaine – and it gave me a job.'

'I stayed with Sue the whole time, even got in the water pool with her in my clothes – she was shouting out to me at the end, so I didn't even wait to get undressed, just kicked off my shoes. When Thomas was born I felt like it was almost a joint effort. There's never been another feeling like it.'

The decision to share the mother's pain is probably a totally unconscious one. The pain which results may be called psychosomatic (pain felt physically, but which has its origin in the mind rather than in actual trauma or injury). Some unsympathetic people dismiss any pain which originates in the mind as not really hurting at all. But in fact it can be just as distressing as pains which have a physical cause – in the same way that symptoms such as stomach pains/nausea/diarrhoea due to serious pre-exam nerves can be just as debilitating as those caused by a virus.

Either way, it seems as though couvade deserves more credibility than it is getting. And that for some men it is an important part of the birth of their baby which is too often being dismissed.

WHAT DOES YOUR BABY FEEL WHILE IT IS BEING BORN?

When a mother is in labour, everyone's attention is focused on what she is feeling. But what about the baby, squeezed by the strong contractions of the walls of what has been its peaceful home for the last 40 weeks? How does he or she feel when being pushed slowly down the birth canal?

As it is not possible to ask the babies themselves, and it has always been assumed by most people that babies do not remember being born so you cannot ask them when they grow up either, no one really knows the answer to this. However, there is a clinical journal entirely devoted to this very area called *The Journal of Pre and Perinatal Psychology*. Amongst its readers and those who submit their research to be published in it, there are many specialists who can make an educated guess. They range from experts in fetal medicine who take a scientific approach, to rebirthing therapists who help people solve psychological problems through reliving birth, and to pre- or perinatal psychologists who are interested in babies' behaviour in the womb and soon after they are born. Despite their very different backgrounds and approaches, they are beginning to come to the same conclusion: that babies surely must feel their birth – and it is probably uncomfortable.

'A baby being squeezed in the uterus when it contracts, and

then down the birth canal itself may well be a painful event. You know how it feels when a doctor puts a blood-pressure cuff on you to take a reading? It might be like having one wrapped around your entire body, squeezing for 30 seconds or so every three to four minutes,' suggests one of Britain's foremost specialists in fetal medicine, Professor Nicholas Fisk of the Institute of Obstetrics at Queen Charlotte's Hospital, London.

'The fetus, including the brain and nerve system, is well developed long before birth, as you can see from caesarean birth of premature infants. It is obvious that labour and delivery are overwhelming and exhausting events for the baby,' says Dr Lennart Righard, consultant paediatrician at the University of Lund and Malmo General Hospital in Sweden.

'We cannot know this for sure. No one can. But there are two schools of thought about unborn babies and their sensitivity to pain,' explains Professor Fisk:

1. That pain is an unpleasant *emotional* sensation in response to tissue damage, and that you need memory to understand and register it *as* pain. Since fetuses can have no memory as such, they can react to stimuli but cannot feel what we would call pain.

We all accept that babies in the womb do indeed react to touch and pain stimuli. Our research looking at the level of stress hormones which they release when a needle is placed in their liver to deliver a vital prenatal blood transfusion tells us this. You can measure the sudden upsurge of stress and injury hormones in their systems, as it shoots up to six times their usual levels of endorphins and twice the level of cortisol. But can you call this 'feeling pain'? Other experiments have shown that plants react physically when uprooted – yet few accept that this means they feel pain as such.

2. There is another school of thought that unborn babies may well feel pain as adults understand it. And most doctors would now accept that newborns certainly do.

However, this is relatively new thinking. Ten years ago

the newborns who needed an emergency cardiac operation would be given open heart surgery without anaesthetic. This would now be thought barbaric, as we know – again from checking the level of stress hormones present in their bloodstream when they underwent such an operation – that they were indeed in great pain. It also became obvious that the newborn babies who had anaesthetics for operations recovered far better than those who had no anaesthetic.

If babies feel pain while their mother is in labour, we will have to try and find a way to ease this. But it is very difficult to give an unborn baby painkillers. If you administer them via the mother it would completely knock her out and may even affect some of the baby's vital functions such as their breathing. We are able to spray anaesthetic on babies' heads if we need to attach a monitoring clip to it or take a blood sample from there during labour, but so far that is all.

'Physiologically, the neural structures required for pain perception are well developed and active in late pregnancy, as are the neurochemical systems associated with pain' writes Jan Nijhuis, assistant professor in obstetrics and gynaecology at the University Hospital of Nijmegen in the Netherlands. 'Fetuses respond to touch on their lips at seven weeks . . . perhaps prenatal sensory experience may serve as a running-in period for the sensory systems.'

Some say it is sentimental to think that babies might suffer when they are being born – and that it is irrelevant whether they do or not because they cannot remember it afterwards. However, Peter Hepper, Professor of Psychology at Queens University in Belfast has recently reported that a fetus can remember more than is generally thought. In 1992, for example, he carried out a study which showed that babies whose mothers regularly watched the TV soap opera *Neighbours* when pregnant would react to its theme tune for weeks after they were born. He is currently setting up a Fetal Behaviour Centre at Queens University in Belfast to 'examine the fetus's sensory perceptions and learning abilities, which could tell us a great deal about its future growth and development'. His team has recently found that unborn babies exhibit the ability to learn as early as 24 weeks, and they feel it may be able to do so even earlier.

'Whether an unborn baby feels pain or not is very difficult to determine as pain is so subjective – and it is all too easy to anthropomorphize fetal behaviour as if they were a fully fledged adult,' says Professor Hepper. 'All we can say is that everything is functioning from a physical point of view which would enable it to feel pain.'

WHAT CAN BE DONE TO PREVENT BABIES FEELING PAIN?

If babies do feel pain when they are being born, there is plenty that can be done to help. Although medical science has not yet found a way to give unborn babies painkilling drugs, there are other ways of reducing any discomfort they may be feeling, based on the idea that much of what helps a mother during labour will also help her baby. There are two important approaches to this:

1 Avoiding mechanical problems in labour: A labour that does not take too long and proceeds without problems is less likely to be uncomfortable for the baby than one where they get stuck and have to experience long periods of ineffective maternal pushing or many long hours of being squeezed by contractions.

But both you, your midwife, obstetrician, your partner and any other helpers can, and do, all work together to help ensure that you have as smooth, uncomplicated and swift a birth as possible.

2 Helping the mother remain as relaxed and calm as possible: It has long been argued that unborn babies are aware of many of their mother's strong emotions and that if she remains calm, they will too. If, however, the mother becomes very anxious, nervous or upset, her stress hormones will be carried across the placenta to the baby who may also begin to show signs of distress.

> Most of the self-help techniques practised by mothers to
> help ease any pain and encourage labour progress smoothly
> – breathing, relaxation, visualization, self-hypnosis, warm
> baths and aromatherapy – tend to have a calming effect
> which will benefit the baby as well.

The first to suggest such a strong link between the state of
mind of a mother and her unborn baby was probably Caraka, the
Indian doctor, writing in 1,000 BC. The ancient Chinese were
also convinced of this, so much so that they held prenatal clinics
to help keep pregnant women tranquil. Empedocles also supported the theory that the development of the baby from embryo
stage could be influenced by its mother's mental state.

There are now several modern clinical studies of fetal behaviour
which support the idea that if the mother is alarmed the unborn
baby will be too, and what soothes the mother is likely to also
soothe the baby. And if the anxiety heightens pain for the baby
as it does for the mother, soothing that anxiety will be important
in reducing the amount of discomfort a baby might feel during
its own birth.

Dr Valman of Northwick Park Hospital in London showed in
the *British Medical Journal* that if a mother was anxious, the fetus
increased its level of sharp kicks and squirming movements by up
to ten times. Another (rather cruel) experiment was done by an
Austrian obstetrician Dr Emil Reinhold. A series of pregnant
women was each placed in a relaxed position and monitored by
a scanner. He then told the woman that her baby was not moving.
In every case this alarmed the women so much that within a
matter of a few seconds, their fetuses were kicking furiously.

This does not surprise Roy Ridgway, former editor of the
British Medical Association's *News Review* and *New Doctor* maga-
zine, and consultant to the International Society for Pre and
Perinatal Psychology and Medicine:

> The baby is a human being and feels everything we feel.
> The only thing it cannot do is express them. It is only able

to react in a physical way – by movement, an increased output of stress-related hormones or, if it has been born, by crying.

Its sense of touch is the first one to develop and you can see half-formed fetuses in the womb sucking their thumbs (possibly for comfort, as they do after they have been born). I think that what they feel when their mother is in labour is a great sense of squeezing or crushing in wave after wave of constriction.

From talking to many psychologists specializing in helping small children who are deeply disturbed, I also believe this is where adult fears of enclosed spaces may originate, and why small children like crawling under beds and sofas or making small, dark, enclosed dens under bedclothes.

I do not think normal births are especially traumatic for babies because the majority of children seem to be fine – despite most of them having to be born in the usual, seemingly painful way. But problematic births which were very long or difficult, where perhaps the baby became stuck for some time or needed forceps to pull it free by its head, may be. A mother's anxiety, if it is prolonged, may affect the baby and research suggests that these children may become disturbed later on in their lives.

I even have some confused memories of what I think must be my own birth and they distressed me greatly when I was a child. I used to have a recurring nightmare that I was in a frightening, dark, churning maelstrom of some sort, that I was being sucked into it but that I was a part of it and could not separate myself from it or pull away. According to my mother I was a very large baby indeed, she had a difficult birth with me, and I was stuck on the way out for part of the time.

Ridgway is not the only person who has such memories. Most people believe that birth would be way too far back for anyone to be able to remember, and in ordinary circumstances this is generally true. However, under therapeutic guidance using a variety of methods from hypnosis and mind-altering drugs to different types of psychological therapy, it seems that many people can rediscover memories of their births, and that these memories do on occasion involve discomfort, even pain.

Dr Lennart Righard, who has done some personal research into hypnosis, also reports that he has relived his own birth 'in order to get an idea of what it is like'.

> I think you would feel the contractions around your body at intervals, the pressure around your head and finally the pressure on your chest when passing through the birth canal. To emerge into an entirely new dimension is an over-whelming experience. After this you need to rest – you are very sensitive to what is happening to you, and in great need of love and soft, smooth handling. This is probably the reason why a bath of water has a calming, relaxing effect on a newborn baby. The mother's abdomen is a good place to be, too: warm and smooth with her familiar heartbeats to listen to.

Though there is considerable evidence to suggest that birth memories can be recovered, much of what is said about rebirthing is probably guru-hype. And the other problem is that there is a phenomenon called the False Memory Syndrome where people vividly imagine events which they could swear happened to them. Nevertheless, many researchers are convinced that birth memories, and memories from the womb, can be both recalled and recovered using drugs or hypnosis.

The first therapist to use mind-altering drugs to help people uncover their forgotten birth experiences was a Czechoslovakian psychiatrist called Dr Stanislav Grof who worked in Prague in the 1950s. He became very interested in the effects of LSD as a therapeutic agent and carried out ten years of controlled scientific research on it in Austria, where at that time LSD was freely available for therapeutic purposes. However, when Grof was invited to America in 1967 to take part in a similar research project in Baltimore, he found that thanks to the psychedelic revolution and the powerful youth culture that went with it, the country was in the grip of anti-LSD hysteria. As a result of this he had to continue his work at a lower profile, but in 1975 the wealth of material from his LSD therapy sessions with patients was collated into a book called *Realms of the Human Unconscious*.

The book contains several hundred interviews with patients, many of whom, under the influence of LSD, said they could remember their own births and the physical sensations, including discomfort, that accompanied them. He divided them into four stages of birth which he called the Basic Perinatal Matrices. They range from a tension-free state of calm euphoria to outright terror. The following are some of the themes which recurred most frequently:

- Bliss, calm, a sense of freedom in which to make oneself comfortable, to kick and push. Gorf thought that these memories tended to correspond with being safely in the womb before the birth process began.

- The contractions and shrinking of the enclosing womb during the first stage of labour. This corresponded with a feeling of 'there is no way out', a sense of helplessness, being stuck. Grof called this the 'No Exit' feeling.

- Being pushed down through the birth canal. Interviewees spoke of a 'titanic struggle', culminating sometimes in enormous ecstasy and sometimes in a death/rebirth struggle.

- The delivery. Described in terms of 'enormous decompression', 'expansions of space', visions of gigantic halls, radiant light and colour – which were sometimes interrupted by a sharp pain in the navel, being unable to breathe, gagging, and fearing dying.

Some psychotherapists today use rebirthing and regression techniques to take their patients right back to the moment of their birth (and before) because they feel the event can in some cases have a bearing on some of the psychological difficulties they experience later in life. Many report comments from their own patients sound very similar to the ones from Grof's LSD sessions.

One school of therapy which uses this is called Primal Therapy.

It was devised in the 1960s by Dr Arthur Janov, a now world-famous psychologist formerly with the Psychiatric Department of the Los Angeles Children's Hospital and State of California Narcotic Outpatient Program. According to primal therapist Franklin Wenham who was trained at Janov's Primal Institute in California, a difficult birth can mean that children may grow up into adults who then have difficulties based on what happened to them during labour.

> For instance if someone became stuck in the birth canal, they may well experience becoming stuck at various developmental stages of their life too, trying to repeat the experience until it is resolved. Primal therapy tries to help people relive such early experiences so they are able to understand why they are behaving as they do and can try to change it.

Often, as the person is regressing they will use the voice they used when they were young. First their vocabulary will change to use words that young children rather than adults would use, then they might begin to talk in a toddler's lisp, going further back into baby talk and finally a baby's cry.

According to Mr Wenham, 'The different birth experiences clients have acted out when I was with them have included feeling trapped, in panic, fearing they were going to die because they could not breathe, being enclosed, pressure against or all around their head, and pain (possibly due to compression) in various parts of their body.'

And the first few minutes of life? This too is based on educated guesswork and extrapolation from the little that is known for sure, ie that babies being born are sufficiently developed neurologically to feel pain (the real question seems to be a matter of *when* they begin using them). However, most paediatricians would agree that a newborn baby has no way of blocking out all the sensory stimuli and information that comes rushing at them after birth.

The environment of an unborn baby could scarcely be more different from the one it is born into. In the uterus, it is in a soft, padded, dark environment kept at a constant comfortable temperature. It can hear noises – the gurgling and rumblings of the mother's intestinal tract, the thump of her heartbeat. It can hear some outside sounds too and will jump at the sound of a car backfiring or door slamming nearby. In fact, the womb can be a noisy place, with sound levels peaking at 90 decibels.

But a fetus experiences no rough touches and it is as close to its mother as it is possible to be. So it is not unreasonable to assume that it would be an unpleasant shock for the baby to suddenly find itself in a bright room, being handled firmly by the birth attendants (this may be uncomfortable too as no one has ever actually touched him before) having its reflexes briskly checked and being wrapped in what may feel, after the softness of amniotic fluid and membrane sac, like the prickliest of cloth. And even worse, no mother. No wonder newborn babies, if offered their mother's breast straight after birth, fasten on it gratefully for oral comfort and contact with the soft skin of her chest, along with the renewed security of being gently held.

Further, if the recollections of patients in regression therapy are anything to go by, the newborn's sensations would be even more disconcerting (the choking feeling of being unable to breathe mentioned by Dr Grof's patients) if there were any respiratory problems.

> 'Being born must be like suddenly being thrust from sleeping in a feather bed in a warm, dim room to driving in an MG at 140mph eating a highly spiced vindaloo, listening to Wagner at full volume and having sexual intercourse at the same time . . . only more so. It is the most massive amount of stimuli to crash into the brain at once in the child's entire life.'
>
> *Professor Geoffrey Chamberlain*

THE POSITIVE SIDE OF PAIN

If birth can be uncomfortable or painful for babies as well as their mothers, it seems extraordinary that evolution has allowed things to turn out in this way. But Professor Fisk suggests that the stress hormones babies release when they are being born, possibly stimulated by the rhythmical squeezing of the uterine muscles and birth canal, have a vital biological function which is important for their survival when they reach the outside world. 'They help to stimulate the baby's lungs to work, and complete their maturing. This is why babies born by caesarean have a greater likelihood of initial breathing problems, and often need some help.'

The possibility of babies feeling pain as they are born has, potentially, enormous implications for the future management of obstetric anaesthesia. Pain-relief methods for the mother in labour are currently judged on how effective they are at blocking *her* pain whilst having the minimum possible effect on the baby. Perhaps in the future new methods will be developed which also try to offer the baby pain relief, but without affecting its breathing and heart rate and metabolism.

ADVANCE MEASURES TO HELP AVOID EPISIOTOMY

Episiotomy is a cut made through the skin and muscle of the area between your vagina and anus. It is carried out on about half all women in labour, and though it is intended to provide more room for the baby's head to descend, whether it is done unnecessarily or not in many cases remains a subject of heated debate. It is also something most women would prefer to avoid if possible. Advance self-help measures may help reduce tearing or over-stretching in the perineal area. They may also help avoid the need for an episiotomy:

Massaging your perineum with oil: This should be done daily in the weeks leading up to the birth. Cold-pressed olive oil and wheat germ oil (available from larger supermarkets and health shops) are both good choices as they are rich and thick. Gently stretch the perineum area between your fingers as you rub in the oil for about five minutes or so a day.

How to massage your perineum:

(a) Slide your thumb gently inside your vagina against its back wall.

(b) With your forefinger on the perineum (feel the thick ridge of muscle next to your vagina, just before your anus), massage gently, trying to stretch the vaginal opening.

(c) Try increasing gradually the number of fingers you can place inside your vagina, progressively stretching the skin.

You can either do this yourself or ask your partner to do it for you.

Traditional societies have always had many different techniques for softening the perineum during childbirth. One very common one is to steam or bathe the area just before the onset of labour or very early on in labour. The Buganda women in Uganda sit regularly in a shallow bath of herb infusions in their last few weeks of pregnancy to relax the perineal tissues. Sudanese women steam their genital area by squatting carefully over a pot of herbs that has just been boiled. Moroccan mothers-to-be used to wash their vulvas every day with hot salted water throughout the whole of their pregnancy, and often had regular steam baths to try and keep these tissues supple. The Michoacán Mexican women use the slippery, moist flesh of a prickly pear cactus fruit called nopal to oil the perineum just before birth; the Fang tribe in Africa use a smooth sap mixture, and women in Japan, India and Thailand use oil (often a rich coconut oil).

Pelvic floor exercises: Do as many as you can, especially the part when you release the muscles in your vagina after pulling them up, throughout the whole of your pregnancy. They strengthen the entire area, including your perineal muscles. (See pp. 285–9 for the most effective way to do them.)

Visualization exercises: Try seeing your perineum and vagina in your mind's eye as being soft and stretching easily.

Check your hospital's record on episiotomies: Most deliveries are done by midwives, who would also be responsible for making an episiotomy if they felt it was necessary. However, episiotomies are done more often at some hospitals than others. If you are planning to have your baby in hospital, you could check its episiotomy rates by asking:

(i)   the consultant you are booked with

(ii) your local Community Health Council, whose job it is to monitor all aspects of hospital practice within your area, including maternity care

(iii) the Director of Midwifery Services at the hospital; ask them about the episiotomy rates of their midwifery team.

You could also try casually asking a more junior member of the consultant's firm, perhaps while having an antenatal check-up with them.

According to the charity Healthrights which monitors hospitals' practices countrywide (especially their maternity care), some consultants, and the team of more junior doctors under them, are more likely to carry out episiotomies than others. The reason is often, but not always, that they practise at major hospitals which look after a larger percentage of more problematic pregnancies and so forceps or vacuum extraction is needed. Hence these births may well have had more need for an episiotomy anyway. Sometimes it is more a reflection of the policies of the obstetricians or midwives in charge.

Make a birthplan: This will be a written record of your wishes for your consultant and it will remain in your folder of maternity notes for the midwife who will be with you during your labour to read. Say that you have very strong feelings about episiotomy – and that you do not want one unless it is absolutely medically necessary.

Consider giving birth in a squatting position: Many people feel that certain birthing positions, especially any variant of squatting, may help avoid episiotomy and tearing. Getting into an upright or semi-upright squatting (not just a sitting) position, supported by your midwife and partner, may help you to work with the medical staff to deliver your baby in a controlled and gentle way that will be less likely to leave a tear or make an episiotomy necessary.

There are no clinical trials to prove that this actually does reduce the risk of tears or the need for episiotomies. But there are no studies which show it does not help either, so most childbirth professionals feel that if a woman in labour is comfortable in this position, there is no reason to interfere. Many will actively encourage variants of squatting because they believe it is definitely useful.

In support of squatting, a study of 427 first-time mothers carried out at Milton Keynes Hospital in 1988 using a special soft, low seat, the Gardosi Birth Cushion, which allows women to sit in a supported squat, found that there were a third fewer than expected perineal tears.

According to the Royal College of Midwives: 'Squatting positions are apparently helpful for reducing the need for episiotomy and the likelihood of tears. But we need to start collecting proper data to make sure of this.'

Few women can squat comfortably for long periods unless they have had a good deal of yoga practice and have developed very strong thigh muscles. Check out your local yoga and natural birthing groups (usually run by the NCT and Active Birth Movement – see **Resources**) for help and practical advice on squatting birth positions. Discuss it with your midwife in an antenatal appointment. You may find it comfortable to squat supported by your partner and/or midwife, perhaps placing a cushion under each heel if you cannot get them flat on the floor easily. Ask if the hospital has a birth cushion, as this also puts you in this position without any strain on your leg muscles.

Supporting the perineum: Protecting the perineum with gentle but firm counterpressure as the baby's head is pushing against it is a traditional way to try and help prevent tears. It may help if your midwife supports your perineum with her hand as the baby's head crowns. Crowning comes towards the end of labour when the baby's head is pushing its way past the perineum so you can see it appearing as a widening domed circle. A large study by the National Perinatal Epidemiology Unit is currently under way to find out for sure whether this is effective.

Judith Goldsmith, who has done extensive research into birth in tribal societies, writes in *Childbirth Wisdom*: 'In central Africa the mother sat, knees flexed, on an animal skin set over a deep layer of dry sand that sloped away from a pair of stakes. The sand moulded itself to the woman's body, and being well pressed down in front, might almost be said to support the perineum.' She adds: 'Because in nearly all tribal societies the perineum was close to the ground, it was usually supported by sand, or a skin, or a pile of leaves or even just by the hard earth. This probably helped restrain the baby's head from being pushed out too suddenly.'

Consider giving birth in water: Water birth enthusiasts like Dr Yehudi Gordon and natural birth pioneer Janet Balaskas say that giving birth in warm water helps reduce the need for an episiotomy. This may be because the warmth of the water softens the perineal tissues and makes them stretch more easily.

Ask for hot compresses: Holding comfortingly hot compresses against the perineal area during the second stage of labour can also help the tissues relax and stretch more. If your midwife has time, ask her if she can do this. In case she hasn't, take a clean flannel into the labour ward with you anyway, so you can ask your partner to keep soaking it in hot water, then wringing it out so you or they can hold it against the area.

PAIN RELIEF DURING
CHILDBIRTH

Pain Relief: The Options

The pain relief method you use is a matter of personal choice, necessity, and what's available. And contrary to what some purists may suggest, giving birth to your baby is a major personal achievement whether you get through labour without any form of pain relief – or end up needing to use the strongest drugs available.

BEING BRAVE IN LABOUR

Giving birth without pain relief is not a question of bravery, no matter what others may imply. It is more to do with how you and your body react to labour, and how smoothly the birth is progressing.

There are many other factors involved apart from maternal endurance. Some are physical, such as your own personal tolerance of pain, your reaction to painkilling drugs, and whether the labour is being artificially accelerated (see p. 76). Others are psychological, such as confidence, knowledge, and an ability to relax deeply.

Childbirth can be an extraordinary and wonderful experience if your body is able to adapt naturally and easily to it. Some women report a truly sensual involvement in the ebb and flow of labour's physical effort, especially if they are immersed in water for the birth.

But though every childbirth is special and exciting in different ways for nearly all mothers, sensuality and sheer enjoyment of the way their body is working is not the experience most women report. And it is very demoralizing to be told that you have somehow not done as well as you could because you found you needed strong pain relief.

Unfortunately, in postnatal classes where women often com-

pare notes on their own birth experiences, there can be a certain
amount of competitiveness ('What I went through'). It is not that
unusual to hear one woman saying to another, only half-joking:
'Oh, you weren't one of those women who had an epidural were
you? I did it all with breathing and massage.' It is even more
common to have this implied rather than said, which can be
almost as crushing: 'You had morphine? Oh.'

Mothers going through labour, especially if it is proving very
painful for them, are still seen by some traditional societies as
female warriors whose bravery far outshines that of men. The
Huron of Ontario, for instance, say that a woman proves her
courage in childbirth in the same way as a man proves his in battle.
Every woman does this in her own way whether she belongs to
a tribe in New Guinea or has lived in central Manchester all her
life. Feeling you ought to go through a difficult labour without
pain relief has been likened to making yourself undergo painful
dental treatment without local anaesthetic – unnecessary, and very
unpleasant.

'Women are not cowards', as one woman supporting the cam-
paign for pain relief in labour for upper and working class alike,
wrote in the 1930s. They want the best for their babies and the
overwhelming majority would not want their choice of pain relief
to have even the smallest adverse effect on their child. They also
have every right to ask for – and get – all possible help giving
birth, if they feel they need it. This help includes not only support
and encouragement from midwives and partners, but also the
option of choosing from a wide range of safe and effective
methods of pain relief the one which is right for them.

KEEPING AN OPEN MIND

No matter how much careful thought you give the matter beforehand, you cannot be sure how you are going to feel while you
are giving birth (especially if it's your first baby) until you are
actually doing it.

A study by St Thomas's Hospital in 1987 of women expecting
their first babies found that the number who asked for an epidural

during labour was four times the number who had intended to do so from the start.

Another survey of 106 women who were pregnant with their first child found that 69 per cent of those who expressed any preference at all said they did not want to have any pain relief, or that they just wanted to use TENS or Entonox. Only 12 per cent had already made up their minds to have an epidural. However, when they actually went into labour, 3 per cent had no pain relief at all, 14 per cent used TENS or Entonox, and 60 per cent (many of whom had tried other methods first) went on to have an epidural.

These research findings – and the experience of other mothers – suggest that it's not a bad idea for the plans you make about your labour to have an element of flexibility built into them. They also give some indication as to how difficult it can be to know in advance just what labour might be like for you.

You are less likely to need additional pain relief if you are fully informed about how labour works, have had some preparation in the form of relaxation classes and exercise, and are feeling naturally more confident because of this. However, though classes, preparation and practice can increase the likelihood of a more fulfilling, easier labour without the need for drugs they do not guarantee it.

'At the time the birth is actually going on, your options may be very different to the ones you originally chose, therefore mothers might feel guilty or depressed afterwards when they do not cope with the pain the way they had hoped to.'

'I think the important thing about pain relief is to have all the options open and to be able to select the right one for you at the right time.'

'It is almost impossible to make the right personal decision about pain relief before experiencing complete labour. Before then you just don't know what to expect. This is my second labour and I knew what choices I wanted to make. Knowledge is the key.'

A partner's view: 'After a prolonged labour my partner needed to have an epidural. The psychological effect of having one after months of NCT classes advocating the "Natural Birth" – coupled with my partner's expectations – left her feeling a failure. A great deal of counselling was needed to avoid her becoming depressed.'

DON'T FEEL GUILTY ABOUT ANY OF YOUR DECISIONS

No one but you knows what it really feels like for you personally when you are in labour, so who is to say you should not ask for whatever you need? Every woman gets through her labour the best way she can and anything that helps is welcome – providing there is no medical reason why a particular drug or method should not be used.

Women who had hoped to give birth without the help of analgesic drugs are sometimes made to feel guilty if they later find relaxation, breathing, or immersion in water are not doing the trick and they need some form of pain relief after all. This is unrealistic and unfair, because every woman and every labour is different. And whilst 10 per cent of women are said to be conscious of major physical effort rather than pain in their labours, this is not so for the other 90 per cent, some of whom may find that gentler pain-relief methods are simply not enough.

To make an informed decision about pain relief in labour, women need:

- To be informed beforehand of all the relevant facts about the pros and cons of the different types of labour analgesia (both for their babies and themselves). Only then will they be able to balance this information against the degree of pain they are in, and make their own informed decision about whether to use whatever stronger drugs are available.

- To be assured that strong pharmacological methods of pain relief are there if and when they feel they need them.

- To be supported and encouraged in their choice of the pain-relief method that they feel would suit them, as long as there are no medical contraindications against it. This applies whether their choice is an orthodox method like an epidural, or a complementary medicine such as self-hypnosis.

- Not to be encouraged to have anything at all if they say they do not want it.

It would be exceptionally sad if all the support and encouragement women now have to give birth without unnecessary pain should turn into pressure, whether from friends or natural birthing groups, to refuse all pain relief no matter how difficult a labour becomes.

This is one of the reasons it is very useful to make a birthplan (see pp. 7–10) and discuss it with your carers beforehand. If you find you are coming under pressure from others while you are in labour to have pain relief you do not want, ask your partner to produce your birthplan – a copy of which should already be in your medical notes anyway – so they can speak up on your behalf. No matter how assertive you usually are, it is not always easy to be so in childbirth.

If you feel you want pain relief and others are suggesting that this somehow shows a lack of substance, take no notice; enlist your partner's help with making sure you get what you need. Bear in mind that a strong belief that analgesia is totally unnecessary as long as you breathe properly, relax, use self-hypnosis or other natural methods such as acupuncture or water immersion, is both confidence-boosting and supportive for the women these methods suit. But it is not helpful for women who need more. It can make them feel inadequate and obliged to experience a great deal of unnecessary pain.

Why others may insist strong pain relief is not necessary

1. The experience of the estimated 10 per cent of women for whom childbirth is not painful as such, merely a major physical effort.

2. Most women (including the ones attending, and teaching, your ante- and postnatal groups) appear to forget just how painful their own labours were.

   In 1982 Queen Charlotte's Maternity Hospital in London carried out a survey of 1,000 women and found that of those women judged at the time of their labour to be in severe pain, more than 90 per cent 'viewed the experience with satisfaction in retrospect', which means they felt it wasn't so bad after all, looking back on it.

3. The fact that different women have, physiologically, different levels of tolerance to pain (see p. 40). This means that some women will not be too distressed by a particular level of pain stimulus, whereas others will be.

Different people have different reactions to painkilling drugs, so some mothers will require higher doses than others to achieve an acceptable level of pain control. Don't be put off by those who know no better and assume that asking for extra pain control means you're not as brave as those who get by on the standard dose: 'One painkilling injection is fine for everyone else. How can you say you want more? Don't make such a fuss . . .'

It is easier to make a choice you are happy with both during and after labour if you have as much information as possible about all the pain-relief methods which exist, from the most widely used to the more obscure. The standard information leaflets you may be given at hospital or GP clinics are a good start but they do not tell you the half of what you need to know on all the possible methods. Nor do antenatal classes, because they do need to cover a lot of other ground as well.

For instance, it is helpful to know not only how effective a method is and how it works but when you might be told that you cannot have it, what its side effects on you and your baby may be, how to get it, how quickly it takes effect and how long it can last.

Pharmacological Methods (Drugs)

This chapter deals with the most common forms of pharmacological pain relief used for childbirth and will hopefully answer
many of the questions you might have. The next chapter looks
at all the possible natural (non-drug) methods. Please also see
Resources (pp. 300–318) for additional information.

EPIDURALS

WHAT IS IT?

An epidural is designed to prevent pain signals being transmitted
from your uterus to your brain by blocking the nerves before they
join the spinal cord.

HOW DOES IT WORK?

By delivering local anaesthetic, usually put in at about waist level,
into the fluid inside the spinal sac via a catheter. This used to
mean that you were confined to your bed during labour, but in
some hospital units there are now ambulant epidurals available.
These allow you to retain movement and feeling in your legs so
you can get up, change position, and even walk around a little.

The method was pioneered by a German anaesthetist called
Stoeckel during the early 1900s. However, it developed slowly
in Britain and did not really become popular until the late 60s –
partly thanks to campaigning by female journalists that it should
be freely available.

Nowadays nearly 1 in 5 of women countrywide use it, though
in the bigger hospitals this probably goes up to nearer a third. It

is most popular with first-time mothers; twice as many of them use it as do women who have had a baby before. This may be because subsequent labours tend to be shorter and less painful. It is also popular with women who have had their labours artificially accelerated or induced with a drip, as this can make contractions much more painful than those resulting from a natural labour. Women report that induced/accelerated contractions seem to start far more abruptly so they have little time to prepare themselves; the pains also feel much sharper and occur more closely together than normal contractions.

HOW EFFECTIVE IS IT?

For some mothers it can remove all pain (it can also, if used in sufficient doses, remove all feeling from the lower part of your body). In the 1993 NBT survey, 75 per cent of women said it gave very good total pain relief, and another 18 per cent said it was 'good'.

But epidurals are not necessarily effective for everyone. The NBT survey found that about 5 per cent of women said they were of little or no help at all.

There are a number of reasons for this:

- the dose might be set deliberately low – perhaps because the woman in labour has said she would like to retain some sensation;
- the epidural has been allowed to wear off for the second stage of labour, so the mother will feel when her contractions are starting and so work with them to help push the baby out into the world;
- the epidural has missed an area. Very occasionally it will even anaesthetize the left part of the body but not the right, or vice versa, or you may feel pain in your perineum but none in your abdomen and back;
- as a result of your particular reaction to the drugs delivered via the epidural.

If there is an area which is still hurting, tell the midwife to ask the anaesthetist to come back and have another look at the epidural. It may be that it has not been quite correctly positioned; some anaesthetists are more experienced than others. Even after an anaesthetist has given 100 or so epidurals, they may still need to re-do them sometimes. Estimates as to how often this may happen range from once in every 100 times to once in every 30.

Be insistent about having something done to ease your pain, especially if your labour is being accelerated with drugs with a drip, as this means it will hurt more. Or ask your partner to make a fuss on your behalf. It may be helpful to arrange between you in advance what you will do if this happens (see p. 75)

HOW IS IT GIVEN?

Epidurals are given by an anaesthetist – obstetricians and mid-wives cannot do them for you.

A hollow needle containing a catheter is inserted carefully into a gap called the epidural space (see fig. 6). This is the gap between the bony walls of the spinal canal and the fluid-filled protective membrane sac (the dura) which holds the spinal cord. The space is filled with a loosely distributed type of fat, and blood vessels.

The tube is then taped to your back so it cannot move, and led up over your shoulder. Anaesthetic (such as Bupivacaine or a mixture of local anaesthetics and painkilling drugs) is then injected in liquid form down this tube. More can be added at intervals, usually every two hours or so, as necessary. At some centres, however, it is now more usual to have a continuous infusion of epidural drugs which supplies a continuous level of pain relief, which rarely needs topping up.

A specially trained midwife can do top-ups for the anaesthetist, which is an advantage as you do not have to locate the latter each time you need some more. This is especially important as anaesthetists may be shared with another local hospital (especially for night duty). This means they might not be at your hospital when you need them and, if they are busy with something else,

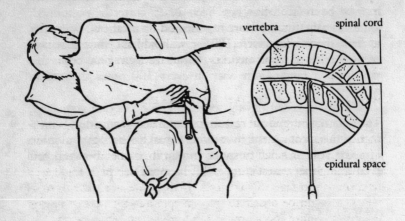

vertebra   spinal cord

epidural space

Epidurals can, at best, give complete pain relief from the waist
down. A local anaesthetic is injected into the space surrounding
your spinal cord.

it could take some time before they can be contacted, and even
longer before they can come back to you.

WHEN CAN I HAVE AN EPIDURAL?

If you are going to deliver your baby vaginally, an epidural cannot
be given until labour is well established, ie your contractions are
strong, regular, frequent (every 5–10 minutes), and beginning
to be painful. Some women experience quite painful contractions
which stop and start for a day or two before real labour begins.
If these were mistaken for true labour and you had an epidural,
you could end up having to stay connected up to the monitoring
and epidural equipment in your hospital bed, with a midwife and
anaesthetist in attendance, for several days.

Epidurals are frequently used for planned caesarean sections.
About 13–14 per cent of babies born in Britain are delivered by
caesarean at the moment. However, less than half of these are

planned in advance. The remainder are unplanned, emergency operations – when a faster-acting spinal or a general anaesthetic may be given (see below, pp. 119–20).

Once an epidural catheter has been set up it can also be used to anaesthetize you for a forceps delivery, should this prove necessary, or for stitches to repair any cuts or tears from a vaginal birth.

WHEN CAN'T I HAVE AN EPIDURAL?

The commonest general reason for not having an epidural anaesthetic is a lack of anaesthetists. If a woman has her baby at home, in a GP unit or small hospital, they will not be available. And even though an anaesthetist might be available, there could be a temporary shortage of midwives. If there are not enough midwives, it might be unsafe to start an epidural, for women having epidurals require special midwifery care in the labour ward.

The commonest medical reason for not being allowed an epidural is a tendency for the woman to bleed. This happens in rare medical conditions such as abruption of the placenta (a bleed into the uterine muscle). An epidural is also contraindicated for a woman taking anticoagulants to prevent clotting defects; she too has a tendency to bleed. It would be wrong to have an epidural if there was any local infection in the region of the back, such as a boil.

An epidural could be complicated if the woman has a low blood pressure, or, paradoxically, if she has a very high blood pressure from pre-eclampsia. In both these cases a very skilled anaesthetist would be needed.

You cannot have an epidural if the labour is already too far advanced, as it might not have time to take effect. It's not possible to have an epidural for a home birth either.

HOW QUICKLY DOES IT WORK?

An epidural takes approximately 20 minutes to set up, and about another 10 minutes to start working. First, however, an anaesthetist must be found – which can take anything from 10 minutes to a couple of hours. This means it will be 40 minutes at the absolute minimum from the time you ask for it until the pain relief sets in – and possibly as much as two or three hours. This may not sound very much, but if you are in a lot of pain it can seem like a very long time indeed.

HOW LONG DOES IT LAST?

Depending on how much local anaesthetic you are given, the painkilling effects of an epidural wear off after a few hours. Top-ups are therefore necessary. Alternatively, the anaesthetist may give you a continuous infusion of the drug so that the effect lasts as long as you need it.

After delivery, it can take several hours for an epidural to wear off fully, so your legs may feel very shaky the first time you get out of bed and someone should be on hand to help you.

If you have had a caesarean section under epidural you will be given a relatively large dose of local anaesthetic. The pain relief will last for about four hours but for some time after this your legs may feel heavy and passing water may be difficult.

A new practice where caesarean deliveries are concerned, according to Dr David Bogod, obstetric anaesthetist at Nottingham City Hospital and secretary of the Obstetric Anaesthetists Association, is to give a very small amount of morphine via the epidural – plus Volterol, another common painkilling drug, via suppository. This carries you through the next couple of days, by which time all you need is paracetamol.

Pros

- Provides the best pain relief of all available methods. In the NBT's survey 75 per cent of the women rated it as very good. Some women said they felt no pain at all.

- Some studies suggest that epidural babies are in a better state than non-epidural babies. Provided the mother's blood pressure is not allowed to drop, the supply of oxygen across the placenta will be better and steadier than it would had the mother been in pain.

- It helps reduce the physical stress of labour, which should cut down the level of stress-related hormones in both your system and the baby's. If you are in less pain, this helps reduce anxiety and any anxiety-related hormones which could, again, cross the placenta and affect the baby.

- Avoids the need for general anaesthetic if you are having a caesarean, so you will not have to be unconscious during the birth.

- Your mind remains completely clear, and you remain awake to enjoy the experience of your baby being born.

- If it is necessary to help the baby out with vacuum extraction or forceps, this can be done relatively painlessly.

- It is helpful for women with high blood pressure. Mothers who have developed pre-eclampsia (very high blood pressure) may be advised to have an epidural but this would need a very experienced anaesthetist.

- If you are giving birth to twins, the second twin to be born sometimes has problems. For instance there may be a delay between the two deliveries, and the delivery of the second may be more complicated. An epidural tends to prevent deterioration in the second baby's condition during the delay. It also makes it less uncomfortable if an obstetrician has to intervene to assist the delivery of either baby.

'I found it a great source of comfort and reassurance to know that when I couldn't cope with the pain any more, an epidural was available fast and successfully. It's just a shame this method has to be associated with so much inter-vention, such as a drip and monitors.'

'Having had an anaesthetic for my first caesarean birth I found the epidural a definite improvement as I was able to be awake for the birth of my second child. It was a wonder-ful experience.'

Cons

- There is no absolute guarantee that you can have an epidural when the time comes, even if you say you would like one well in advance (see **How do I get one?**, pp. 88–9).

- With traditional types of epidural you must remain in bed, either lying on your side or propped up in a reclining position. Having to remain in the same position for several hours and then give birth in that position can be uncomfortable in itself, making you feel very stiff and sore (see p. 87). The new mobile epidurals (see p. 90) mean you can still move about a certain amount.

- An epidural can make it difficult for you to feel and work with your contractions. However, if you are wired up to a monitor you can see them coming on the graph. If there is no monitor, your midwife can sit with her hand on your abdomen and tell you when the contraction is beginning, so you can push with it.

- Some experts say it can make the second (pushing) stage longer. However, this can be corrected with a continuous infusion of oxytocin during the second stage. (There is no good evidence to suggest an epidural is likely to make the *first* stage of labour, when the cervix dilates to allow the baby's head to pass through, last any longer than usual.)

- It increases the likelihood of an assisted delivery (ie when the obstetrician uses forceps or the gentler vacuum method to help pull your baby out) especially if it is your first child (see pp. 84–5).

- Some studies suggest that an epidural can make a baby jumpier for a few days, though this has not yet been conclusively proved.

- If the mother's blood pressure drops the oxygen supply to the baby may be reduced, causing it problems. An epidural can cause this, so it needs to be watched for and corrected if necessary.

- There is controversy over whether an epidural will make you more prone to back problems in the months (or even years) after you have had your baby (see pp. 86–7).

- Some women find the idea of a needle going into their spine upsetting. Many report that the sensation itself, even after a local anaesthetic, is unpleasant – others say they felt nothing at all.

- The procedure is difficult – anaesthetists don't always get it right first time, in which case you'll still feel pain. The painkilling effects can wear off if it's not topped up regularly.

If the anaesthetist puts the needle in at the wrong place, accidentally puncturing one of the membranes protecting the spinal cord, it is called a dural puncture. This does not happen often – according to Dr Bogod the chances are about 1 in 100, but when it does, some of the fluid inside these membranes leaks out, causing a drop in pressure around the head. This pressure drop can produce severe headaches, migraines or neckache.

Usually these symptoms resolve themselves within 24–48 hours after the birth, but the first day or two of trying to bond with your baby can be far more difficult if you also have a debilitating migraine. There have also been rare cases of the problem lasting far longer than that. Out of 74 cases reported in a St Thomas's Hospital study, 23 said they had neckache afterwards but all of these said this persisted for more than a year. This sort of headache needs the attention of an anaesthetist. Do not try and soldier on if you have one.

'The feeling of numbness was good for the pain, but also quite alarming. The epidural also slowed up labour quite considerably.'
'I am not quite sure why midwives are against epidurals, but I think that the potential extended labour time may have something to do with it.'

Does an epidural make an assisted delivery more likely?

Many women who have an epidural go on to have an assisted delivery. This may be because:

- You often can't *feel* when it's time to push. You'll either be told when by the midwife, or you'll have to watch for cues on a monitor screen wired up to your abdomen.

- The epidural itself reduces your output of the hormone oxytocin, which encourages your womb to contract and push the baby down the birth canal.

- The midwife may call the obstetrician to do a forceps delivery because she feels that the second stage of labour has been going on for too long.

Some obstetricians, however, argue that the connection between epidurals and assisted deliveries has been misinterpreted. They say that few women decide before they go into labour that they definitely want an epidural. Usually the decision is made when a woman finds her labour is proving far more painful, more difficult, or more tiring than she had expected. In many cases, women having more difficult births are perhaps the ones who would have needed intervention anyway, whether they had had an epidural or not.

The National Birthday Trust's 1990 survey of women using epidurals showed that 46 per cent of first-time mothers and 58 per cent of mothers who had had babies before gave birth without additional intervention.

According to Felicity Reynolds, Professor of Obstetric Anaesthesia (the only one in the country) at St Thomas' Hospital in London, an epidural need not mean a forceps delivery and there are four ways in which medical staff can cut down your chances of needing one:

1. Top up your epidural if necessary at the beginning of the second stage, rather than letting it wear off. An epidural infusion must be tailored to your needs and may need to be slowed down.

2. Let your baby's head descend well, encouraging you not to push until then.

3. Provide an oxytocin drip.

4. Be **patient**.

Some obstetricians want to intervene after an hour and a half to two hours of pushing. This may be necessary if the mother is exhausted. However, if she feels she can continue (and provided the baby is not in any distress) she can be encouraged to do so for anything up to three hours (Kader and Campbell 1986), and so have more chance of avoiding a forceps or vacuum delivery (Studd *et al* 1980).

Fear of a risk of paralysis

Some women feel very wary of an injection to their spinal area: 'It's the one awful thought that flashes through your mind just as they are putting the needle in: "What if it should paralyse me?" Like when you have a general anaesthetic – it occurs to you: "What if I'm not out properly and they start to operate?"'

There have been occasional stories of this happening, often described in loving detail by tabloid newspapers. Even if you only heard it third or fourth hand, it is still the sort of thing that would stay at the back of anyone's mind because it is so very alarming. However the chances of it happening are extremely rare – Jason Gardosi, consultant obstetrician at Nottingham University Hospital, puts them at 'literally, one in a million'.

But even though the chances are remote, it is a good reason for *only* having an epidural in a maternity unit which has experienced anaesthetists on 24-hour call – because should the drug enter the spinal fluid it can cause ascending paralysis and eventual cessation of breathing. During one of your antenatal appointments, check if your hospital offers 24-hour anaesthetist cover.

Epidural-related back problems

There has been a good deal of work, both by hospitals such as the Royal Birmingham Maternity Hospital and individuals such as natural childbirth campaigner and anthropologist Sheila Kitzinger, to suggest that an epidural can virtually double your chances of developing back problems later on.

Professionals like osteopaths and chiropractors who work with musculoskeletal problems and specialize in treating back disorders also feel, because of the female patients they see, that there is a link:

> Amongst the women who have come to see me with back trouble following childbirth, I would say that a disproportionately high percentage of them have had epidurals.
>
> *Susan Moore, past president of the*
> *British Chiropractic Association (1987–93)*

> I have run ante- and postnatal back clinics for women for many years, often seeing the same mothers both before and after they have had their babies. The clinics do not just treat pregnancy and childbirth-related back problems, they are there to prevent them too and help keep the women's backs healthy.
>
> From what I have seen, I cannot help feeling there is a link. But searching through all the published medical papers on the subject, it's still hard to come to a definite conclusion – most suggest a connection then say that more work is needed in the area.
>
> *Stephen Sandler, Director of the mother and baby clinics at*
> *the British School of Osteopathy*

A study carried out in Birmingham in 1989 examined women who had given birth both to first and subsequent babies up to nine years before, and concluded that an epidural increased their chances of back problems afterwards from 10 per cent to 18 per cent.

St Thomas' Hospital in London also did a study of 1,000

first-time mothers who had epidurals, and got similar results: 11 per cent of those who had not had an epidural and 17 per cent of those who had complained of backache after they had their babies. However, according to Professor Reynolds, only half of these were new backaches. The rest had already developed back trouble during their pregnancy. She adds:

> And I am not sure that the backaches concerned were usually that bad. We offered treatment to everyone who said they had this problem, but only 100 made an appointment to come and see us and only 30 actually turned up.
>
> We also did another study to see if the drugs used in the epidural were causing muscle weakness and creating back difficulties that way, yet it appeared to make no difference. It seems as if it is more to do with the position the woman is sitting in during labour. I would often come in to see how they were getting on, to find they had initially been propped up in bed then had slipped downwards. This left a gap large enough to get my hand through between their back and the angled back of the bedframe which was meant to be supporting it.
>
> The other thing is that women who have a caesarean section with an epidural do not complain of post-delivery backache. This also suggests that the sitting position has something to do with post-epidural backache.

How to stay comfortable when you have an epidural

To get around the problems of aching back muscles because you are lying or sitting for so long in one position (especially if you can still feel some contraction pains) or post-epidural backache Professor Reynolds suggests that you or your partner ask the midwife to:

- Tilt the foot of your bed up a little to help stop you from slipping down

- Keep checking that you have not slipped down (you always do if you are sitting there for hours)
- Prop you up again to combat this
- If possible, help you gently and carefully change positions every so often (eg from lying on your side to sitting up, and vice versa)
- Use the hand-through-the-gap-between-bed-and-back test, to check you are constantly supported properly
- If you are propped up, whether it is sideways or facing forwards, check that the bend is at your hips and not your waist
- Massage your neck and shoulders as tension will build up there too, which can give you a cracking headache. (However, some women in labour do not want to be touched much, so this is not comforting for everyone.)

Other positions you might try include:

Being propped up cross-legged in the tailor position

Lying on your side

Sitting propped up with knees slightly bent, a cushion underneath them

Use a beanbag (the hospital may have one, or you can bring in your own for labour) for your lower back support – they can be very comfortable.

HOW DO I GET ONE?

Epidurals are available in about 75 per cent of all hospitals where babies are born. However it is not always possible to have one when you ask for it. In an NBT survey, midwives reported that the most likely reason for this (given by 47 per cent of midwives who took part) was because an anaesthetist was not available. In another 24 per cent of the cases the woman's condition did not permit the use of an epidural. For 10 per cent of cases the delivery unit was too busy to set up and supervise another epidural. Inadequate staffing (a midwife needs to stay with you if you have an epidural) was the stumbling block in 6 per cent of cases, and in a further 3 per cent the baby's condition was the problem.

So, much depends on whether there is an anaesthetist available to set it up and enough midwives to look after you. In fact, small cottage hospitals which care for fewer than 2,500 maternity cases a year may not be able to keep skilled anaesthetists on a 24-hour duty rota because this requires a minimum staff of four anaesthetists. Even if you put it in your birthplan that you would definitely like an epidural, and agree this with your obstetrician and midwife beforehand, there is no absolute guarantee that it will be possible when the time comes – and they should make this clear to you. If you would like an epidural, always check whether it is available 24 hours a day.

The midwife needs to be in almost constant attendance for an epidural birth – to check your blood pressure, monitor the baby, etc. Some units do not have enough staff to permit this kind of one to one care.

To be told: 'We are very sorry, but we simply don't have anyone available to do it at the moment,' can be devastating to a woman whose labour is proving very painful, over-long or exhausting. The only way to guarantee that an epidural will be available is to go private and pay for *all* your pregnancy, birth and postnatal care – and for a private anaesthetist. Generally, you cannot have free NHS care for everything else and then pay privately for the anaesthetist alone. And even if you do opt for private medicine, outside the Greater London area there is still a small chance that your private anaesthetist may be on another case when you need them.

An obstetric care package can cost between £2,000 and £6,000, depending on which obstetrician looks after you and where you live. A private anaesthetist will cost several hundred pounds. Private room charges can be as high as £400 a night (which could add up to more than your actual medical care if it is your first baby and you find you need to stay in for several days).

MOBILE (WALKABOUT) EPIDURALS

This is a new type of epidural which has been developed at some hospitals in the UK. The traditional type works by blocking all the nerves from the site of the injection downwards, so the lower abdomen, pubic area, thighs and legs are all numbed. In the majority of cases this will either obliterate or greatly reduce pain from your womb contractions. Unfortunately it also means you need to go through the rest of your labour lying down or reclining; walking will be out of the question because your legs will be wobbly at best, if not totally unusable.

Mobile epidurals work slightly differently in that the mother has a combination injection (into the same place as for an ordinary epidural) of either a weaker form of local anaesthetic than for a normal epidural, and a pethidine-related drug which allows good pain relief without the usual high dose of local anaesthetic, which makes moving your legs so difficult. This should mean that any contraction pains are blocked out but you can still use your legs to move about.

In a recent study at Queen Charlotte's Hospital in London, 300 women tried this new form of epidural, and over half of them either walked around or sat in a rocking chair for some part of the labour. Side effects included itching for 17 per cent of the women (but it was only 3 per cent of cases were severe enough to need treatment). Because they were able to walk to the toilet to pass water, there was no need to have catheters inserted into their bladders as they would have done with the traditional type.

At the time of writing, many more babies have been born using this type of anaesthetic – another 2,000 at Queen Charlotte's, and several thousand more at other hospitals which are now trying this form of pain relief for labour.

GENERAL ANAESTHETIC

WHAT IS IT?

An anaesthetic which produces complete unconsciousness.

HOW EFFECTIVE IS IT?

Very. If the anaesthetic used is sufficient – which it almost always is – you should be completely unconscious throughout (see below: waking).

HOW IS IT GIVEN?

The anaesthetic is usually given through a plastic cannula at the back of the mother's hand. It goes directly into her bloodstream, which is why it works so fast. At this stage the anaesthetist will be pressing against the cricoid area of the mother's neck to stop any of the acid contents of her stomach reaching the lungs and damaging them.

Next, the anaesthetist will give another injection to relax the muscles. A tube will then be passed down her throat and into the windpipe. When this is done, they can stop pressing against the woman's neck. The tube is then linked up to a ventilator which breathes for her during the operation, ensuring she has both the right amount of gas to keep her asleep and the right amount of oxygen for her baby.

WHY MIGHT A GENERAL ANAESTHETIC BE GIVEN?

Reasons include:
- emergency caesarean
- a very difficult forceps delivery. However, if it is thought this is going to be that problematic, the medical staff should discuss the option of a caesarean with you beforehand
- to remove a retained placenta.

WHEN CAN'T I HAVE GENERAL ANAESTHETIC?

Generally you can be guided by the anaesthetist who sees you. Obviously, recent meals may rule it out, but this is rare in labour. It may not be suitable for some women with severe heart or respiration problems.

HOW QUICKLY DOES IT WORK?

Within a few seconds of being administered.

HOW LONG DOES IT LAST?

As long as the operation lasts. Depending on how much is used, you could be awake very soon after the operation is over.

Pros

- Can enable invasive but life-saving procedures for the mother, baby, or both to be carried out almost immediately when necessary.

- Total pain relief

- Works very fast.

Cons

- Women who have had a caesarean birth under GA may feel disappointed and distressed afterwards. Some report feeling that they were not there at all, that they have no real way of being sure the baby is theirs, that they have missed something very important and precious – awareness of their baby's birth. Others say that they felt very disappointed they were unable to give birth to their child naturally. If you feel you would like someone to talk to about this, or any other aspect of caesarean birth, such as how to be up and about as fast as possible afterwards or the easiest ways to breastfeed, contact the Caesarean Support Network (see Resources).

- If the procedure needs to be carried out as a sudden emergency, this can be very alarming indeed for both the woman and her partner.

- There is a risk of infection and thrombosis.

- Both mother and baby may be sleepy, nauseous, or groggy for some hours afterwards, which can lead to difficulty in bonding together, and in establishing breastfeeding.

- The GA may affect the baby's ability to breathe unaided, and it may need additional help.

- Adults usually recover from most of the effects of a GA within 24 to 48 hours. However it can take weeks to recover totally and some people report feeling more tired and lethargic than usual, and with less mental sharpness, for a few weeks after even minor surgical procedures under GA, such as a laparoscopy.

- The effects of a GA birth on the baby remain a subject of heated debate. Conventional advice suggests that your baby should show no ill effects after 24–48 hours. However, some mothers report that babies born under GA seem irritable, less responsive generally than expected, and want to suckle for only short periods until they are several weeks old which can make establishing breastfeeding more difficult.

Waking up during a caesarean section under general anaesthetic

Everyone has heard stories of people waking up on the operating table in great pain, unable to let the medical staff know, and suffering enormous distress both during and after the operation. This is more likely during a caesarean than during any other sort of operation as the anaesthesia is kept lighter at the beginning until the baby has been lifted from its mother's womb so the anaesthetic drugs affect it as little as possible. Once the baby is out, the dosage is then increased.

Having said this, awareness under a general anaesthetic for caesarean section occurs *very* rarely. But it does happen. It is estimated[1] that around 200 of the 40,000 mothers who have the operation under general anaesthetic each year* in the UK experience a degree of consciousness at some point during the procedure.

However, this awareness seldom takes the form of pain. It is far more likely to be an awareness of:

* According to Edinburgh consultant D. B. Scott, as reported in *Anaesthesia*, Vol. 46, p. 674.

- being physically manipulated
- hearing noises like their baby crying, the ticking of anaesthetic machinery, or snatches of the medical staff's conversations

- They may also have a memory of dreaming.

A study carried out by St James' Hospital in Leeds in 1991 shows that this is happening less now because anaesthetists are increasingly customizing doses of anaesthetic drugs rather than sticking to rigid guidelines. As a result they report that (at St James' at least) the number of women who said they could remember dreaming under anaesthetic for caesarean-section dropped from 8.6 per cent in 1983 to 3.7 per cent in 1989, and those who said they had at least a fleeting degree of awareness under anaesthetic dropped from 1.3 per cent in 1983 to 0.7 per cent in 1988. Encouragingly, of the 3,000 women they questioned soon after their caesarean, none said they could remember any pain.

But the fact remains that very occasionally a woman can wake while having a caesarean under GA. In 1988 Margaret Ackers went to court over her own experience of this and became the first woman to win compensation for it, plus, perhaps more importantly, public acknowledgement of what had happened to her. Too often, says the Caesarean Support Network, women who wake under GA are told they were imagining things, when what they really need is prompt, sympathetic counselling – and an explanation.

As a result of the Ms Ackers case, other women have since followed her lead and anaesthetists have been actively looking at further ways of reducing this risk.

MEPTAZINOL

WHAT IS IT?

Also known as Meptid, it is a similar type of drug to pethidine. Seldom used for childbirth.

HOW EFFECTIVE IS IT?

About the same as pethidine.

HOW DOES IT WORK?

Meptazinol acts in two ways:

1. By altering the chemical action of certain cells in the brain, to increase analgesic effect.
2. Binding on to the opiate receptors in your brain and stimulating them in the same way as an opiate drug like morphine would.

HOW IS IT GIVEN?

It can be given to you by injection, but the best way to have it is in a diluted dose delivery system that is under your own control – you can regulate it yourself as and when you feel you need to using a simple hand-held control. This means *you* decide how much you need and when, but there is also a device built in to the system to prevent overdosing.

Meptid also exists in tablet form, but this is not very helpful for women in labour.

WHEN CAN I HAVE MEPTAZINOL?

At any time throughout your labour.

WHEN CAN'T I HAVE MEPTAZINOL?

There are no specific contraindications to the use of this analgesia. However, the problems occurring with pethidine may happen to a lesser degree (see pp. 111–13).

HOW QUICKLY DOES IT WORK?

Within 15 minutes of being injected into you, hitting its peak about 60 minutes later.

HOW LONG DOES IT LAST?

Altogether it lasts for three to four hours.

Pros

- Under your own control.
- A reasonably effective form of pain relief.
- Can be used at any time during labour.
- Affects the baby less than pethidine does.

Cons

(side effects)

- You need to remain in one place to use it (though you can lean over cushions or beanbags on a bed to get more comfortable if someone helps you into position).
- May make you feel drowsy, dizzy, or sick. About 5 per cent of women report nausea, though it's less likely to make you feel sick if you only have a little of it. Other side effects are similar to those you get with pethidine (see pp. 111–13).

HOW DO I GET IT?

It is available in most obstetric units in Britain, but only a small number of women use it. In the 1993 NBT survey 1.8 per cent said they had had it. This may well be because few are told it is available.

* According the findings of Nicholas and Robson '82, Jackson and Robson '83.

NITROUS OXIDE AND OXYGEN

WHAT IS IT?

A gas, known colloquially as gas and air. Often called by its brand name Entonox which is a mixture of oxygen and nitrous oxide. When you breathe it in, it helps dull pain.

HOW EFFECTIVE IS IT?

In the 1993 NBT survey, 84 per cent of women described the pain relief it gave them as being 'good' or 'very good'. This contradicts several earlier studies which had suggested that its pain-relieving powers were no better than a placebo (dummy treatment) though in many cases, even placebos can have a pretty good effect.

HOW DOES IT WORK?

It works by depressing all the activities in the central nervous system of the brain. It also affects the nerve endings in your spinal cord, reducing their ability to transmit pain signals.

For some people, breathing only 20 per cent nitrous oxide may produce mild pain relief with slight sedation and general impairment of feeling, but most need higher concentrations. It is usually used at 50:50 concentration for women in labour, and can produce reasonably good pain relief – plus a feeling of detachment, described as similar to having drunk two or three double gins. You may also feel slightly dizzy and have mild amnesia afterwards.

HOW IS IT GIVEN?

The gas may be piped to your bedside or it may be stored in a cylinder on wheels (see fig. 7), so it can be moved easily to wherever you are when you want to use it – reclining on your bed, sitting, leaning over a chair, big cushion or beanbag, resting

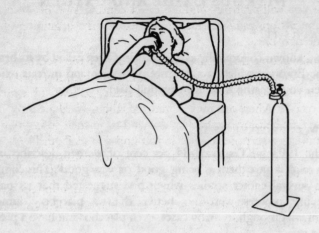

You use nitrous oxide by breathing it in through a rubber mask. The mixture of gases is either piped to an outlet on the wall above your bed, or it may be in a wheeled cylinder placed next to you.

against your partner as you squat on the floor. When not actually breathing in the gas you can move from place to place between contractions, but you must not walk about or stand while actually inhaling it as it can make you feel dizzy.

The gas cylinder is connected to a mouthpiece which you either hold between your teeth or through a mask fed via a fat, corrugated rubber tube. To use it, just breathe in through the mouthpiece, which you hold to your face yourself. There is a demand valve on the cylinder so the gas only starts flowing through when you breathe in. You can also breathe out through the mask or mouthpiece.

Tips on using it

- Because the gas has a slightly delayed effect, use it as soon as you feel a contraction beginning rather than waiting until it really hurts – that way the gas will be having its full effect by the time the contraction hits its peak.

- Only take four or five deep breaths of the gas per contraction, or you will probably find the effect continues on between contractions as well, causing you to miss the beginning of the next one.

- Some people do not like the smell (despite the fact that anaesthetists insist the gas is odourless), which has been described as sweetish, and slightly sickly. So have a breath or two of it when you look round the labour ward a couple of months before your baby is due and try it then so it will not come as a surprise to you. If you find you really dislike it, you can discuss other forms of pain relief with staff, before you need them. Many women who did not like the smell to begin with, however, say that this became unimportant to them as their labour progressed and their contractions started becoming stronger.

'I didn't like the smell at all and thought I wouldn't use gas after all. But when the contractions really started and my midwife suggested I try some again, I found I forgot all about the smell as I was so pleased to be able to take the edge off the pain.'

'It really gave me something positive and helpful to actually *do* during the contractions instead of just wait until they had gone away.'

'I think gas and air [sic] should be tried before things get out of hand so you know how to use it and how it makes you feel.'

WHEN CAN I HAVE NITROUS OXIDE?

Almost any time you like, but it is generally used towards the end of the first stage, when the contractions are strong, rather than very early on when many women wish to be moving around.

Some midwives prefer to keep it for when labour has 'become well established', because if you use Entonox for a very long time it can make you feel sick or dizzy.

It can be used when you are actually delivering your baby. However, some obstetricians feel this distracts you from the effort of pushing your baby out and prevents you from doing so as quickly or as efficiently as if you had no pain relief at all. Discuss this with your obstetrician and midwife beforehand. Should they advise you against it but you find when the time comes that you cannot manage without it, provided there is no medical reason why you should not have it, keep using the Entonox. You are the one having the baby and the pain – not your birth attendants.

Other occasions when nitrous oxide might be used include very rapid deliveries where there is not really enough time to use any of the other methods, and as analgesia for any stitches to repair a tear or episiotomy cut after your baby has been born.

It may also be given when the midwife or doctor wants to do a vaginal examination to see how far your cervix has dilated so they can tell how close you are to delivering your baby. These examinations are done regularly throughout your labour and can be uncomfortable (though not as a rule painful as long as you can relax while they are being done) because you will be very sensitive in that area during childbirth. The examinations may be less uncomfortable if your midwife carries them out while you are lying on your left side, rather than flat on your back. This is also better for the baby as it helps maintain a good blood supply to the placenta.

Nitrous oxide can also be used to supplement an epidural which is wearing off.

WHEN CAN'T I HAVE NITROUS OXIDE?

The modern equipment for giving nitrous oxide and oxygen depends upon the mother holding the mask to her face and taking deep enough breaths to open the valve to allow the gas to flow.

Hence, if she is drowsy or not fully conscious, she should not be given nitrous oxide and oxygen. Nor is it wise for somebody else, such as her partner or the midwife, to hold the mask to her face, for that would also mean she could not regulate the gas supply any longer.

Contractions need to be well established (regular and fairly strong) before you start taking it, so gas can not be used in the very early stages of labour.

It is not a good idea to use the gas continuously for several hours on end, as there is a very small risk it would have a slight effect on baby due to the mother over-breathing.

HOW QUICKLY DOES IT WORK?

After two or three breaths.

HOW LONG DOES IT LAST?

It is absorbed rapidly through the lungs, enters the blood swiftly and is carried to all the body's tissues. After you stop breathing it in, it is expelled from the body almost as quickly so you need to keep using it to retain its pain relieving effect.

If taken for a long period, it can make some women feel rather drunk for about 20 minutes after they stop using it.

Pros

• It is under your own control, so whenever you feel you need some more you just breathe it in. Because you control the mask or mouthpiece yourself, you are unlikely to get an overdose.

• Widely available.

• It can be effective, and though it does not provide complete pain relief it will at least take the edge off.

• You can stop and start using it as necessary with almost instant results.

- Can use it at any stage of your labour, including, should you need stitches afterwards, when these are being done.

- Can be used when there is no time for any other method to work or to be set up.

- You can keep on moving about a certain amount (ie around your room or cubicle rather than up and down the hospital corridors) between breaths of Entonox, as long as you sit down well supported while inhaling it. You can also get into different positions (leaning over a beanbag or the back of chair, supported squatting) which will help your labour.

- You can use other forms of pain relief with it. These include all the self-help and natural methods: yoga, self-hypnosis, breathing and relaxation, Autogenic Training, massage, and visualization. Many midwives would let you use it in water pools and baths (not showers, in case you were to feel groggy and slip over) though some water birth purists would say that the water itself should be sufficient (and for many women, it is). TENS does not interfere with Entonox and there is no reason why you should not use both at once.

- It can be used if you are having a home birth.

- Available in ambulances, so you can use it if you need to go to hospital in the middle of your labour.

- Can be used during vaginal examinations, which are done periodically throughout your labour to see how far your cervix has dilated.

- Can be used while waiting for an epidural – worth knowing as the delay between requesting an epidural and feeling its effects can be at least an half hour, usually more (see p. 79).

- You can also use Entonox at the same time as an epidural, should the epidural not be doing a very good job of pain relief for you because it has missed an area or has been allowed to wear off a bit in the second stage of labour so you can push better.

'Gas and oxygen has two effects: first the anaesthetic effect and, secondly, it helped her concentrate on breathing to provide some distraction.' *(A partner's view)*

'It went well with the breathing methods of relaxation I had been taught in my antenatal classes – gave them extra power.'

'I thought it wasn't making much difference, so I stopped using it. Then I realized what a difference it was actually making after all and grabbed the mask back again.'

'I don't think I let go of the mask for my whole labour, and delivery. It was my lifeline and my moral support.'

Cons

- Some women find they do not like the smell of the gas (the smell has been attributed to the rubber of the mask/mouthpiece rather than Entonox itself, though not all women agree with this) especially if they are feeling sick, which is quite common during labour for at least part of the time.

- The baby may be slightly affected if the mother inhales the gas for too long and then finds she is over-breathing (ie breathing rapidly and shallowly) as this can reduce both her own, and therefore her baby's, oxygen supply.

- The nitrous oxide in Entonox can, in theory, cause changes to a particular enzyme which affects the baby's metabolism. In practice, this has never been found to happen to a great enough extent to make any difference.

- Some dizziness and disorientation may occur, especially if you are taking too much of the gas. If this happens, stop for a while, until this passes.

- May produce some measure of amnesia.

> 'Gas and air acts as a distraction from the pain but does not really relieve it.'
>
> 'It smelt disgusting. I was really disappointed because I wanted the least invasive method of pain relief there was, this was it – and I just couldn't bring myself to use it.'

HOW DO I GET IT?

Just ask. In the NBT survey Entonox was found to be available almost everywhere where babies were delivered. It is also carried in ambulances (and the staff on board are trained in its use) should you need to use one to get you to hospital. Most midwives make it available for home births too.

About 75 per cent of all women use it at some point in labour.

PARACERVICAL BLOCK

WHAT IS IT?

Local anaesthetic injected on either side of the cervix.

HOW EFFECTIVE IS IT?

It gives good pain relief.

HOW DOES IT WORK?

It works by numbing the nerves as they leave the uterus and travel with the uterine arteries, towards the side wall of the pelvis. The method was popular some years ago, but is now less frequently used. Can be used for procedures such as forceps delivery.

HOW IS IT GIVEN?

There are usually two injections, one on each side of the cervix (at the 3 o'clock and 9 o'clock positions).

WHEN CAN I HAVE A PARACERVICAL BLOCK?

It would usually be used at the *end* of the first stage of labour, when the dilatation of the cervix may be becoming especially uncomfortable. Its effects last into the second stage of labour.

WHEN CAN'T I HAVE A PARACERVICAL BLOCK?

Early in labour. You can only have it once the cervix has reached at least the 6cm dilation stage.

HOW QUICKLY DOES IT WORK?

Within a few minutes.

HOW LONG DOES IT LAST?

Between 30 and 60 minutes. It cannot be topped up though.

Pros
- Can be effective.
- Very fast acting.
- Fairly easy to perform.

Cons
- Not effective for all stages of labour.
- Does not last very long.
- Could affect the baby's heart rate, causing it to slow. This may either be because of the direct action of the local anaesthetic on the blood vessels supplying the uterus, or those vessels going into spasm a little later on when the local

anaesthetic drug has been absorbed into the mother's bloodstream.

HOW DO I GET IT?

You can ask your midwife or doctor about it. It is not often done now, so they may offer you an alternative instead.

PETHIDINE

WHAT IS IT?

A synthetic, narcotic drug similar to morphine. It is also known as meperidine, Dolantin, Dolosal, and Demerol.

HOW EFFECTIVE IS IT?

In the NBT survey of 1993, about 25 per cent of women said the pain relief they get from pethidine was 'very good', but a further 25 per cent found it of no help at all. Midwives seem to find pethidine is more helpful than the women who use it do. This may be because for 80 per cent of women who use it there is a substantial sedative effect as well. If a woman in labour is making little fuss because she is drowsy (though still in considerable discomfort) an observer might understandably think that she is in less pain than before she was given the pethidine.

HOW DOES IT WORK?

It is a strong painkiller and sedative with a powerful antispasmodic action. However, the dosage used is not high enough to affect the ordinary levels of womb contractions either during the first or second stages of labour, or when you deliver the placenta afterwards. It is helpful if you are having very painful contractions early on in labour.

About 40 per cent of women use it in their labour, according to the 1993 NBT survey.

HOW IS IT GIVEN?

A midwife, or doctor, can prescribe pethidine for you. They will inject it into the muscle of your thigh or buttock.

It may also be given intravenously (injected straight into a vein) in which case it works straight away. However, this is not usual, and it would only be given in this way if you needed to have an emergency procedure that required immediate strong pain relief but did not merit anything like a general anaesthetic, such as an emergency forceps delivery. Not only does the intravenous injection take effect immediately, the drug is also cleared more rapidly from your bloodstream, so it might last for about half an hour then wear off.

You can also have the drug via patient controlled analgesia (PCA) where you administer your own doses via a computer-controlled syringe pump. This is not widely available at the moment.

WHEN CAN I HAVE PETHIDINE?

Many midwives feel that pethidine should be given only in the early stages of labour. Most would refuse to give it to a mother who is only about two hours away from delivering her baby, because if the drug crosses the placenta into the baby's bloodstream it can affect the baby's ability to breathe unaided. This does not matter so much while the baby is in the womb, because it is still attached to the placenta via its umbilical cord and is supplied with food and oxygen dissolved in blood. But once he or she is born, the cord is severed, and the baby will have to breathe for itself. If its breathing mechanisms have been depressed by the pethidine, this may be difficult and help will be needed.

Because it is can be hard for a midwife or obstetrician to be certain how much longer a labour is going to take (for instance, some women can suddenly accelerate very fast after the waters break) most, to be on the safe side, will not give a woman pethidine after her cervix has dilated two thirds to three quarters of the way. The exact cut-off point varies from hospital to hospital and obstetrician to obstetrician. But usually it is reckoned to be after a woman's cervix is 7–8cm dilated (if this is her first baby) or 6–7cm if she has had babies before.

However, contrary to popular belief, Prof. Felicity Reynolds (the only professor of obstetric anaesthesia in the country) says that all the evidence shows that pethidine is more likely to have a longterm effect on the baby if it is given to the mother *early* in her labour, as the drug and its by-products will then have had time to not only cross the placenta into the baby's bloodstream, but to build up in their tissues. It can take several days for this build-up to be eliminated from the baby's system. During this time he or she may seem fretful or unresponsive. On the other hand, if given within an hour of birth, the drug's effect on the baby will be kept to a minimum.

> The effects of pethidine on the baby can be countered by giving the antidote, called naloxone, as soon as it is born. This cannot be given via the mother while the baby is still in the womb because it would cancel any pain-relieving effect the pethidine was having.

WHEN CAN'T I HAVE PETHIDINE?

Pethidine can be a good pain reliever, but it does tend to depress respiration a little. This does not matter in the mother who has established her breathing patterns, but pethidine goes across the placenta and can affect the baby, who has got to start breathing for the first time just after birth. Hence, it is probably unwise to use pethidine if an early labour is taking place as a premature baby may often have breathing difficulties anyway.

Do not use pethidine if you suffer from any of the following:

- acute asthma (the same applies with other morphine-related drugs)
- chronic bronchitis or emphysema

- severe liver disease, as this will prevent your body being able to break down the drug easily

- if you are taking monoamine oxidase inhibitors for depression. About 3 per cent of pregnant women will have some measure of depression and this drug is one of the treatments for it, though it is rarely used now.

- if you are allergic to pethidine.

If you have had pethidine during a previous labour and it did not suit you, there are other pain-relief options which (if available) may have fewer side effects for you and your baby. Discuss the alternatives fully with your midwife, the hospital anaesthetist, and your obstetrician beforehand. The NCT, AIMS and the Active Birth Centre will also have information which may help you (see **Resources**).

HOW QUICKLY DOES IT WORK?

It works within about 15 minutes, usually hitting its peak within 30 minutes.

HOW LONG DOES IT LAST?

A standard pethidine injection would last for about two or three hours for the mother and its after effects may be felt for several days by the baby. During a normal labour, you would have either one or two doses. However, if you only have a very small dose, the effect would be gentler and last for a shorter time – and midwives are now customizing doses for individual women whereas before there was a single standard amount given to all.

Pros

- Pethidine is a mood enhancer, but women's reactions to it are mixed. Some feel euphoric and high, distanced from the pain, as if they were floating above it. Some simply say they felt knocked sideways by it.

- It can make you feel very sleepy. Many women actually fall asleep, despite the contractions. If you are getting tired out, a doze like this for an hour or two can be very helpful and refreshing, enabling you to manage the rest of the labour with renewed energy.

- If your contractions are painful but progress remains slow and your cervix is only dilating extremely gradually, then pethidine may be helpful. Women have often found they were able to sleep or doze for as much as three or four hours after having pethidine, then wake up to find they are in good established labour at last. However, every woman's labour is different and progresses at its own rate. It may be that your labour is just naturally going at a slower rate than most; even though your contractions have yet to open your cervix, they have been making a real difference by softening and thinning the muscle fibres. A soft, ripe cervix will dilate easily when it is ready.

> An apparently non-progressing labour does not necessarily mean that nothing constructive is happening. You may just be in a longer than usual preparation stage, before the action really starts.

- You may find it is far easier to relax after having had pethidine. Reducing stress has many advantages, including a reduction in the pain you feel. Pain is reduced when you are not stressed or frightened (see p. 24 and pp. 49–50).

> 'I think pethidine helped me to relax. It did not actually relieve the pain though. What it did do was make me mentally dopey and out of control and less concerned about it.'
>
> 'I was very disappointed with pethidine as I could not think straight and would not do as I was told.'
>
> 'It was an effective pain reliever but it slowed my contrac-

tions down and made me very drowsy. I'd have been better equipped physically to push without it.'

One woman reports imagining 'lovely trees, bushes, sparrows and squirrels in the room: I think I was flashing back to a long walk my husband took me for on Hampstead Heath the day before. I kept whispering to him that I could see them, making him look at them too – but insisting he promised not to tell the staff in case they thought I was mad.'

Cons

For the mother

- About one in three women say it makes them feel sick. A few may actually vomit. Some women feel very nauseous during their transition phase and are sick anyway, so any sickness caused by the pethidine would be in addition to this. Pethidine is usually given together with anti-sickness drugs. To be on the safe side, it is worth you or your partner checking with the midwife that she is definitely going to give you anti-nausea medication too.

- The sleepiness can have a down side, in that waking up later to find you are suddenly in full-throttle labour can be a shock.

- Slowing labour: the sedative effect can be blamed for slowing the birth down, or as one partner put it: 'Pethidine gave her pain relief but it brought labour to a *standstill*.'

- It can make you feel very unsteady on your legs, so it's probably a good idea to stay in bed after having had pethidine.

- You may feel disorientated by the narcotic effect of the drug. Rather than feeling agreeably high you could feel as though you are unpleasantly drunk and your labour is out of control.

- Even hospitals which allow the mother to eat small amounts during her labour may not do so if the mother has had pethidine.

- Pethidine is not usually given towards the end of labour (despite the fact that this may be the best time for it, from the point of view of not affecting the baby), but if it is, you may later find you have no memory of your baby's birth. This is not usual, but when it happens it can be very upsetting for the mother.

- A small number of women – less than 1 per cent – may suffer severe disorientation and hallucinations. These can be pleasant, like the woman who saw trees and squirrels, or alarming: another woman recalled thinking she was in a prison hospital where one of the doctors was going to take her baby away as soon as it had been born.

- Some women (about 5 per cent) may experience lowered blood pressure. It is important to tell your midwife or doctor *immediately* if you feel any dizziness or tingling in your fingers and toes. Temporary drops in blood pressure can be countered easily if you have a drip for a while.

For the baby

- The baby may be rather sleepy and unresponsive for a few days after its birth, while it is still getting the pethidine out of its system. This may sound as if it's no bad thing – many women hope for a peaceful baby who sleeps a good deal. But unfortunately this sleepiness can also depress the baby's suckling reflex whether it is being given a bottle or a breast, causing problems for women who are trying to breastfeed, especially if they have not done so before. A baby who is sleepy and less alert at first may also be a little more difficult to bond with than a more responsive baby.

  In fact, pethidine's reputation for causing baby drowsiness probably dates back to the days when it was routinely given in larger, set doses – during the 1950s, 1960s and early 1970s. These days it is more often tailored to the needs of the mother and it can be given in doses as low as 25mg at a time.

According to Doris Hare, the President of the American Foundation for Maternal and Child Health, many US midwives only use very small doses at the optimum time.

Sometimes, a midwife will feel it best to only give a very small dose and see how the woman in labour does with this, before giving more. This may well be enough to relax a nervous or worried mother so her labour can progress better.

- Some paediatricians report that such babies may also be more fretful and more easily startled than babies whose mothers did not have pethidine during their labours. Again, this may sound fairly trivial, but a fussy baby who cries a lot and is less willing to be comforted can make its first few days quite difficult for a new mother, who may start losing confidence in herself.

- It may affect the baby's ability to breathe well. This is barely noticeable to the naked eye, but it can certainly affect the baby from the moment it is born. This is another reason why the baby should be given naloxone after a pethidine labour.

HOW DO I GET IT?

Pethidine is available in 97.6 per cent of all labour wards in the UK. Just over a third of all women use it in childbirth.

PUDENDAL BLOCK

WHAT IS IT?

A regional nerve block in the form of an injection of local anaesthetic, usually lignocaine. Overall, nerve blocks are used for 10 to 20 per cent of all births.

HOW EFFECTIVE IS IT?

This varies, because it can only block the major nerves supplying the perineum – not all of them.

HOW DOES IT WORK?

By deadening feeling around the perineum.

HOW IS IT GIVEN?

It is injected into the area just below the pelvis to deaden the nerves which lead into the vulva.

WHEN CAN I HAVE A PUDENDAL BLOCK?

It is frequently used if a baby is being delivered with the aid of forceps or vacuum extraction, especially if it is in a breech (bottom-first) position.

WHEN CAN'T I HAVE A PUDENDAL BLOCK?

There are very few times when local anaesthesia should not be used. A small number of women are allergic to local anaesthetics of this type and they usually know about this. The mother must tell the doctor or midwife about her allergy to a particular local anaesthetic, so it would not be used.

It is only used for delivery, not at any other time.

HOW QUICKLY DOES IT WORK?

It takes effect in a few minutes.

Pros

- Acts quickly.
- Can be most effective.

Cons

- The pudendal nerve is close to the blood vessels which supply the baby in the womb. If very large amounts of anaesthetic are used, this could cause a change in the fetal heart rate, but this is not usual as the person doing the injection will limit the amounts of drug they use.

- Not all women find it effective.

BIRTH BY CAESAREAN SECTION: PROCEDURES AND PAIN RELIEF

A caesarean section is a safe, common – and major – abdominal operation. It involves the obstetrician making an incision through your abdominal wall and then your womb, and lifting your baby out. It may be done under heavy local anaesthetic (an epidural) or light general anaesthetic. The procedure may be planned well in advance for a particular day, or it may need to be done as an emergency procedure.

Caesareans have their own section in this book as they do need specific types of analgesia and anaesthesia, and present different potential recovery problems from ordinary vaginal births (see also pp. 283–99 for post-operative discomfort which may arise and what can be done about them).

PLANNED CAESAREAN SECTIONS

If you are having a baby by planned (elective) caesarean section, you do not need to wait for labour to begin, nor will you experience any labour pains. Instead you will be booked in to hospital to have the operation done on a specific day.

Possible reasons for a planned caesarean include:

Your previous baby or babies were born by caesarean: If you want to have the next baby vaginally, discuss it with the doctor beforehand. About a third of all previous caesareans now go on in later pregnancies to give birth vaginally, so if there is no good medical reason to prevent it (apart from the fact that you had a caesarean last time around, perhaps because the baby was becoming short of oxygen, see below), you could go into labour in the usual way and see how things went. However if problems did develop, the staff would intervene and you would need a repeated caesarean. There is an organization called the Caesarean Support Network which gives information and encouragement to women who have had previous caesarean sections and wish to try and avoid another: see **Resources** for details.

Placenta praevia: This means that the placenta is lying low down in the womb, perhaps right across the opening where the baby would be coming out.

If the baby is lying in an unusual way: This means that some part of the baby other than the front of the head (such as their bottom or feet) is against your cervix, which could make it difficult for them to leave your womb. When a baby is lying with its back across the exit to the womb this is called a transverse lie, and a baby in this position cannot be born vaginally.

Cephalo-pelvic disproportion: This is when the baby's head is too large to allow it to pass through your pelvis easily. Sometimes it is obvious that this is going to be a problem, but at other times the medical staff are not quite sure, and will let you have a trial labour where you go ahead and try to give birth without intervention for a while. If your labour does not progress well and the baby's head is clearly not coming downwards into the birth canal, you would have a caesarean section.

Irregular contractions: Experienced staff should be able to tell the difference between a labour which is naturally very slow but progressing at its own pace, and one which is hardly progressing at all and needs some major help.

Unless the baby was showing signs of distress, or you were exhausted, they would probably try accelerating the labour gently at first perhaps with prostaglandin pessaries, then with an oxytocin drip, before resorting to a caesarean operation.

Certain health problems which you, the mother, may have: These include:

(i)   Active genital herpes (when the herpes sores are actually visible as opposed to when they have disappeared). If your baby is born vaginally when you have an active herpes sore, you can pass the infection on to him or her.

(ii) Diabetes, as this can mean that your baby will be very large.

About 10 per cent of women develop gestational diabetes (diabetes which develops only in pregnancy and disappears again afterwards).

(iii) Very high blood pressure.

(iv) Full blown eclampsia, which may result in convulsions in the mother and the premature birth of her baby.

(v) Being HIV positive. There may be less chance of passing on the infection to your baby during the birth if they are delivered by caesarean.

Some mothers are worried at the thought of being awake for a caesarean operation, or of having an injection into their spine.

If this is the case for you, now is the time to say so, and ask about the option of a general anaesthetic instead. Modern general anaesthetics have fewer side effects on the baby or mother than in the past but it is still safer if you can avoid it. In many hospitals, 80 per cent or more of caesareans are done by epidural. It is vital that you choose the way of having your caesarean section that you feel the most comfortable with, both as it is being done and afterwards.

HOW AN ELECTIVE CAESAREAN IS DONE

If there is time, the staff may prefer to shave your pubic hair so it will not get in the way of the incision. However, unless you are luxuriantly hairy it would be unlikely to obscure the obstetrician's vision anyway, so usually close clipping of the hair is all that is necessary. If there is time to shave the area, there would also be time to clip it and the latter is preferable from your own point of view as shaving increases the risk of infection, and pubic hair can be extremely itchy when it grows back again.

First you might be given a suppository to empty your bladder and bowels, because once the epidural was working you would no longer have any control over either. You would also have a catheter put into your bladder to drain it, and a drip in your arm to help prevent falls in blood pressure.

If time allows you could talk to the obstetrician about where you would prefer the scar to be. The most usual place is a horizontal one just below the bikini line, but there may be medical reasons why they would need to do a vertical one which would reach from your pubic area to your belly button.

If you are having epidural anaesthesia, the equipment would be set up (see pp. 77–79), if not you would have a general anaesthetic (see pp. 90–4).

NOTE: An epidural is not the same as a spinal anaesthetic. A spinal involves actually going through the dura and injecting anaesthetic into the fluid with bathes the spinal cord itself. It is very fast-acting and is therefore used for emergency caesareans (see pp. 119-20).

If the caesarean is done under GA you will wake up remembering nothing about the procedure. Some women feel very uncomfortable about waking up and being handed a baby and told it is theirs. It may help if your partner or one of the staff takes a Polaroid photograph as the baby is being lifted from your womb, if you feel this is something that might worry you.

Where an epidural is used, a screen will be placed across your waist so you cannot easily see the operation. If you do not want to be able to see anything at all, avoid catching any reflection in the overhead mirrored lights above the operating table and concentrate on your partner (if they have remained with you) or on talking to one of the staff instead. However if you would like to watch, the staff can hold a mirror up for you. The doctor would usually carry on an encouraging running commentary for you anyway.

After the incision is made, the amniotic fluid is sucked out (you will hear this as a gurgling or sucking sound), the doctor lifts your baby out, pressing down on your abdomen as they do so. Many women say they experienced a rummaging feeling 'as if someone was doing their washing in my stomach', others report sensations of pulling and stretching. Both you and your partner will be able to see the baby being lifted out and hear the first cry he or she makes. You would then be given an injection to speed up the expulsion of your placenta, and would, if you are awake, be able to hold your baby straight away if you wished, while the incisions are being stitched.

The birth itself takes less than 10 minutes, but the careful sewing up afterwards may take 40 minutes. You do not need any additional pain relief for this because your epidural will still be working.

EMERGENCY CAESAREAN SECTIONS

You may need to have an emergency caesarean operation. This is one which instead of being planned and discussed well in advance, becomes necessary at what may be very short notice, when you are already in labour.

It may be needed for any of the reasons already mentioned above. But one of the most common additional reasons is that the baby is in distress, usually because it is not getting enough oxygen. This can happen as a result of:

- the physical stress that labour places on your baby, as well as on you yourself;
- the umbilical cord, which should carry its supply of oxygen, becoming partly or totally squashed so little or no oxygenated blood can get through;
- the placenta, whose job it is to supply the cord with blood and oxygen, failing to do so because it has peeled away from its position on the womb's wall.

Signs of a baby's distress include a very rapid heartbeat, which can be detected through a fetal monitor device placed on your stomach, and meconium. If your waters have broken and there is some greenish material in them, this is the baby's earliest form of bowel movement and the substance is called meconium. An unborn baby will empty its bowels before it leaves the womb if it is alarmed by lack of oxygen.

Setting up an epidural may cause some delay, so if the baby

needs to be born straight away to avoid harm, you would have a spinal or a general anaesthetic for your caesarean operation (please see pp. 90–94). This means it would only be 10 minutes or so before the operation was done, compared with 30–40 minutes for an epidural.

The exception is if you have already been having an epidural for pain relief during your labour, and the necessary tube already set up. If this is the case, the anaesthetist could use the existing tube to give you a much heavier dose of local anaesthetic, one which would numb you totally from the waist down so you would not feel the operation.

There is a small possibility that an epidural may not work fully, but in almost all cases this becomes very obvious before the operation begins, allowing for an additional method of anaesthesia to be used as well.

(Non-Pharmacological) Natural Pain Relief

A 1990 National Birthday Trust survey of methods of pain relief discovered that women used the following in labour:

Entonox (nitrous oxide)	60	per cent
Pethidine	36.9	per cent
Relaxation and breathing	34	per cent
Epidural	19.3	per cent
Massage	19.3	per cent
TENS	5.5	per cent
General anaesthetic	3.9	per cent
Diamorphine	2.1	per cent
Meptid	1.8	per cent
Homeopathy	0.4	per cent
Hypnosis	0.07	per cent
Acupuncture	0.02	per cent

(no other methods recorded)

This is not necessarily because the majority of women prefer drugs to natural methods. A substantial proportion do use the latter – about one in three uses relaxation/breathing, one in five uses massage, and one in twenty opts for TENS. And although fewer than 1 per cent use complementary therapies like homeopathy, general interest in them is blossoming in the UK and, if recent *Which?* reports are anything to go by, customer satisfaction with them is up at the 80 per cent mark.

There are a number of possible reasons for the fact that pharmacological methods of pain relief are used more than natural methods:

- Pharmacological methods are far more widely available in hospitals than the non-drug methods. For instance, nearly all hospitals offer epidurals and pethidine but a smaller proportion has TENS and only a few offer their own water pools (some will not even let you bring your own in).

- Few people are aware that complementary therapies can be helpful for pain during labour. And if they have heard about this in general, they seldom know which ones, or where to find out further information on the subject.

- If you ask about the methods of pain relief available, you will probably be given printed information on the various drugs on offer and perhaps on relaxation and TENS. But it is a rare hospital unit which will tell you about the all natural methods too because, with a few notable exceptions, they themselves know very little of the subject.

- Pharmacological methods are provided free on the NHS. Whereas, apart from water, TENS machines and relaxation, the non-drug methods usually need to be arranged by the woman herself beforehand – and paid for on a private basis. Not every woman can afford this.

- Drugs are perceived as more powerful methods of killing labour pain; natural therapies are thought to be gentler (and therefore, some would argue, less effective).

- While it is difficult to say in advance how much *any* method of pain relief (drug or natural) is going to help you, in general, natural methods tend to be less predictable than drugs and there is often no way of knowing beforehand how well they will work for you personally. While the same can be said of the drug treatments, it is arguably true to a lesser extent, and statistical records mean that the success/failure rate is easier to put a figure on.

- Far more is known about the side effects of pharmacological drugs in labour than is known about natural methods. There is little published work on the effects of the latter, while professional medical journals have printed a great deal of research into the former. Most doctors, and many mothers, find it reassuring to use methods that are known quantities, ie drugs. On the other hand, what limited research exists would suggest that adverse side effects are far less common with natural and complementary methods, and more likely to be of a minor nature.

Relaxation and breathing is one of the few complementary techniques which is commonly used for labour. This is because it is the most widely available. It is taught in all NCT and active birth classes, and also (in less detail) in most NHS antenatal classes as well. It is very possible that if there was more information available to women on the other complementary therapies, they would grow in popularity.

It is often suggested that it is mostly middle-class women who are interested in natural methods of pain relief. However, a study* of 700 women in six maternity units in south-east England carried out in 1993 showed that class/occupation made no difference. Most women from all classes were keen to avoid painkilling drugs if possible.

Drugs are something the labour ward staff can easily give you. Natural methods (apart from water and TENS) tend be things you have to go out and get for yourself – and often do for yourself as well. For instance, if you want to use homeopathy, acupuncture, breathing, deep relaxation or self-hypnosis, it can involve considerable commitment and involvement on your part.

1 You may need to find – and pay for – a trained therapist to give you the treatment or teach you to apply it yourself (which can often involve extensive practice beforehand).

2 You will need to understand a fair bit about the therapy you select.

3 You may have to work hard to convince your maternity unit that it is a good idea, especially if you want to take a complementary therapist into hospital with you to help with pain relief.

* Josephine Green, *Birth*, Vol. 20, No. 2, pp. 65–72.

HOW TO GET COMPLEMENTARY THERAPY AS PAIN RELIEF FOR LABOUR

Check several months in advance with the Head of Midwifery Services that they are happy to allow this. Not all of them will be. It depends upon the policy of the midwifery unit, and that of the consultant who is responsible for your care.

If they are reluctant, you can try and argue your case. If they refuse outright, try to find a more sympathetic hospital. Community midwives are a good source of information, as they should know what attitude local hospitals and their consultants take towards complementary medicine in the labour ward. It's worth knowing too that different obstetricians in the same hospital will have different policies, and some may be more sympathetic to this type of pain relief than others.

Anaesthetists are usually very approachable and happy to answer questions from pregnant women about all aspects of pain relief. If you would like to talk to one, ask when you are at one of your antenatal appointments. They may also know of one of their colleagues in a nearby hospital who has an interest in complementary medicine, or they may be sympathetic to it themselves and be prepared to have a word with any sceptical consultant obstetricians on your behalf.

Your local Community Health Council (under C in the phone book) may also be able to help as they gather information on all aspects of clinical practice for all the hospitals in your area. Alternatively you could contact AIMS, the NCT, Healthrights (see **Resources**) or ask the therapists themselves. If they have an interest in taking care of pregnant women, they should know of hospital units which have looked kindly on them being present in the past. Some of the more liberally minded hospitals may well be private, which presents a problem unless you have plenty of money (a privately managed pregnancy and birth generally costs between £2,000–£6,000).

WARNING

Do not simply arrive at the hospital in labour with a therapist in tow.

Because some maternity units are not happy about the use of complementary medicine in childbirth, there have been instances when women have arrived with their therapist, only to be told to choose between them and their partner being present at the birth.

This means you would probably have to pay the therapist's usual charge as a cancellation fee, even though you find yourself without your chosen method of pain relief.

There are several reasons why maternity units might object:

1 Some are concerned about the therapist's insurance status should there be complications. Check that your therapist has the necessary professional insurance to cover them to give pain relief to women in labour. Let the hospital know that they have it.

2 The maternity staff may not be well disposed towards complementary medicine in general.

3 Though they are interested in it in theory, they may want to see its safety and effectiveness proved in standard extensive clinical trials before they allow it to be offered on their premises. Unfortunately, few clinical trials involving complementary medicine and its use for analgesia in labour have been translated into English. Most of the clinical trials for acupuncture are written up in Chinese (though the library at the Royal College of Midwives has several references in English on acupuncture and childbirth – see **Resources**). Most of the clinical references for reflexology are in Russian and East European languages. Many of those for aromatherapy are in French. However, there are some in English and at the end of this book there are several references for each therapy, and it may be helpful to quote these in discussions with your midwife or obstetrician.

See *How do I get it?* at the end of each section for advice on how to find a professional therapist or teacher.

BREATHING AND RELAXATION

WHAT ARE THEY?

The more anxious and tense you are, the more something is likely to hurt.

This is because tension, anxiety and fear are key factors in your perception of pain. There is a sound physiological reason for this – anxiety triggers a fall in the level of natural pain-soothing hormones (endorphins) while at the same time causing the body to increase its production of adrenaline-like hormones. (Please also see pp. 46–48).

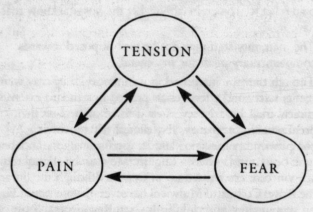

Fear, tension and pain all feed off each other, and can create a vicious circle which is difficult to break. The rationale for education about childbirth is to help women understand, and therefore not be afraid of what is happening. Many natural pain-relief methods for labour, such as breathing, visualization, massage, self-hypnosis, Autogenic Training, also work by helping remove any fear or tension, and so reducing and relieving pain.

In the early 1930s a London doctor called Grantly Dick-Read set about breaking this vicious circle by developing a pioneering regime of antenatal training for women which involved:

1 Teaching expectant mothers about the physiological process of pregnancy and birth so they could understand what was happening to them.

2 Teaching them muscular relaxation techniques to use during labour, which though they took some time to learn could produce a virtual state of hypnosis in certain cases. Women were told they could start using these when they were about 2cm dilated in their first stage, then later to relax deeply in between the strong, expulsive contractions of their second stage.

3. Breathing control. This was based on the techniques of Hatha yoga.

He also encouraged the woman's partner to be involved, lending practical as well as moral support – by massaging her back, for instance. Again this was a revolutionary idea because at that time male partners were strongly discouraged from coming anywhere near a woman in childbirth.

According to Dick-Read, his technique was basically a psychological one of helping women to overcome their fear of childbirth. His methods spread to Western Europe and America, where it was combined with the teachings of a famous French obstetrician called Lamaze. Lamaze also believed in full psychoprophylaxis, a more heavily hypnotism-oriented approach which became very popular in Russia, where some doctors claimed it could give up to 70 per cent of women a pain-free childbirth.

Dick-Read's methods are still used in Britain today, having been developed and simplified by both the NCT and the Active Birth movements.

BREATHING AND RELAXATION

Together with being given full information about what will happen during childbirth, these are two foundation stones of any psychological form of pain relief that you do for yourself. **Any** relaxation technique can be adapted to use in childbirth, including yoga, self-hypnosis, Autogenic Training, and different types of meditation. However, the National Childbirth Trust and the Active Birth movement both teach a straightforward form of breathing control and relaxation in their classes especially for use during labour (both organizations run relaxation and preparation for childbirth classes countrywide – see **Resources** for details).

In the NBT survey 1990, 34 per cent of mothers chose to use relaxation and breathing, making it the third most popular method of all after Entonox and pethidine. However, only 3.8 per cent of midwives recorded that their patients were using it. This may be because the mothers did not mention it and the midwives failed to notice, as breathing and relaxation is usually a fairly quiet, low-key activity.

HOW EFFECTIVE IS IT?

From an effectiveness point of view, 89 per cent of women said they found it either 'very good' (a third) or 'good' (over half).

'The breathing gave me something to concentrate on during my contractions.'

'I blew the pains away as hard as I could each time they came. It was not pain relief as such, but I found that if I did this I could cope OK. This and back massage took me all the way through to the end.'

'I think there is a difference between pain relief and coping with the pain. Relaxation and breathing is a good way of coping, without actually relieving it.' *(A partner's view)*

'It's something that helps, and you can do it yourself, you don't have to ask the midwife to give it to you. This makes all the difference.'

WHAT DO I HAVE TO DO?

Relaxation used as a form of pain relief is not what many people think of as relaxing – perhaps sitting down with your feet up, watching TV and drinking tea. You may not be actually doing anything like cooking, cleaning, working or playing, but your mind is still working and your body may still be tense. Nor is it the same as lying down for a rest, when the body might well be technically at rest but it can still be tense in places, and your mind may be refusing to switch off.

Deep relaxation involves both your body and mind. It could be described as a systematically and deliberately induced state of mental calm, combined with looseness and ease in the body.

Breathing: The quickest way to relax deeply is also the easiest and simplest: change the way you breathe.

Of all the body's involuntary physical processes (those which carry on happening without you consciously thinking about it) breathing is the easiest one to bring under your control. It encourages relaxation because just by breathing slowly and deeply you can alter other aspects of your nervous system too, and gain control over your general levels of tension.

When you are feeling anxious your breathing will be more rapid and shallow. Many naturally nervous people say that most of the time they feel they are only breathing *halfway down*. And if you are in pain, again your breathing will be more rapid and shallow.

But if you can deepen and slow down your breathing you will have a direct effect on the other physical processes of your body such as heart rate and blood pressure, and it will also encourage true deep relaxation. Several forms of yoga and meditation use slow deep breathing to reach altered mental states. In deep meditation an individual might breathe only about four times a minute; those who have trained in the discipline for many years may only breathe two or three times a minute.

ASTHMA

Women who have asthma or had it when they were children often have bad memories of not being able to breathe. They may feel uncomfortable trying to deliberately control their breathing in labour.

If this is a problem for you, and you are going to antenatal classes such as those run by the NCT, let your tutor know. She may be able to suggest some other helpful techniques you can use to relax your body.

In the past, breathing for birth meant practising different styles of breathing at different points in the contraction – deep breathing at the beginning and middle, then shallow panting at the end. However this was not always helpful as some women found this complicated, and others often started their shallow breathing too soon. Steady deep, strong breathing throughout is far simpler.

Practise breathing/relaxation as often as possible, because the more you practise the easier you will find it. Try to set aside 15 or 20 minutes a day which are solely yours. Make sure you are not going to be disturbed: ask your partner to keep any children you may already have out of earshot, unplug the phone if you might be able to hear it when it rings. Perhaps have a warm, soothing bath beforehand, or play a favourite piece of calming music for a few minutes before the actual relaxation practice begins.

Mentally, put any outstanding business and all your worries in a large box or lidded basket, then 'see' yourself shutting it firmly with a lock and key, so it can be opened later and its contents dealt with when your relaxation has finished.

REMEMBER

The more often you do it:

• the easier it will be
• the more quickly you can slip into relaxation mode

- the more deeply you will be able to relax, so that it will be more difficult for outside stimuli such as noise or an unfamiliar environment (like the hospital labour ward) to disturb you
- the more effective it will be as a method of natural pain relief when you are giving birth to your baby

Exercise I: just breathing

The idea of practising breathing may sound unnecessary because we breathe all the time. But breathing, and being aware of *how* you are doing it, are two different things.

Breathing in an ordinary way, without thinking about it, keeps you alive. Being aware of your breath enables you to control it. When you are able to do this – and you may find you can do so very quickly – it can also help you cope with any pain you feel.

1. First, get really comfortable. Wriggle about a bit until you are.
2. Rest your feet on the floor, hands loosely on your lap or thighs, back supported in an upright chair, or lying back in a comfortable armchair. Some women find sitting in the cross-legged tailor or half-lotus position is very comfortable, perhaps with their back supported by a wall.
3. Close your eyes. Or if you prefer to leave them open do not focus on a particular spot – try and develop a blank unfocused stare instead.
4. Just breathe out slowly. This out-breath part of your breathing cycle is the relaxing part: notice how your body starts to let go and loosen as you do it. This is the part you will be concentrating on to release tension and help you cope with the pain.

Exercise II: Relaxing as you breathe

Tensing up and holding your breath is a common, and instinctive, reaction to something hurting. Many women find they do this during labour, and it can mean they then experience more pain than they need to. The following can help you overcome this reaction:

1. Start by breathing as slowly, evenly and deeply as you can. Concentrate on doing this for a while, perhaps 5 or 10 minutes. Let it settle into an easy rhythm.

2. Relax your body, starting with your forehead. Breathe in and frown as you do so – then breathe out, letting the frown go smooth again.

3. Now it's time for the face. Breathe in and scrunch it up, then breathe out and relax it again, letting your lower jaw drop a little so your lips part slightly. Make sure your tongue isn't clamped against the roof of your mouth, or with its tip pushing hard against your front teeth. Feel your face becoming softer and smoother.

4. Next come the shoulders. Breathe in and shrug them up to your ears, at the same time flexing your arms at the elbow and clenching your fists. Breathe out, letting your shoulders drop back down, relaxing your arms and stretching/flexing your fingers and wrists. Do this exercise two or three times if you wish – the shoulders, hands and neck are usually the most tense parts of the body.

5. Breathe in and make your neck as long as you can, then out again, allowing it to sink gently back to its original position.

6. Now for the small of your back. Breathe in and arch gently to stretch the back, then breathe out and let it go. Breathe in again, pulling your shoulder blades in together, stretching your upper back, and then let that go.

7. Breathe in and tighten up your abdominal muscles. Notice what this does to your breathing. Let that breath out again and relax the abdominals.

8. Breathe in and tighten your bottom and pelvic floor. If you are not sure which muscles are the ones in the pelvic floor, they are the ones you would use if you needed to simultaneously stop a bowel movement and hold in a burstingly full bladder.

As you breathe out, let those muscles relax, imagining tension flowing out of you as you do so.

9. Breathing in, tighten your thigh muscles, then relax them as you breathe out. Do the same with your calf muscles.

10. Breathe as you flex your feet upwards towards the ceiling from your ankles, then breathe out and relax them again.

11. Breathe in, curling your toes tightly. Breathe out and let go.

Now just breathe in and out, slowly and deeply for a while, feeling all the tension flow out of your body each time you exhale as you sink gently into a deeper state of relaxation.

This may sound complicated, but all you are really doing is tensing each bit of your body in turn (as you breathe in) and releasing it as you breathe out.

It may also be difficult to do this while trying to read the instructions above. If so, ask a friend to read them in a calm, quiet voice as you follow them, or even put them on tape for yourself.

BREATHING WHEN YOU ARE ACTUALLY IN LABOUR

Some women say they find it helpful to blow, rather than simply release, each breath, as if they were blowing the pain away.

- If the contractions become too strong and you forget to breathe steadily and deeply, don't worry about it. Just breathe the best way you can during it, and use relaxation/deep breathing in the intervals *between* contractions instead.

- Get your partner to help you by breathing in a slow, deep steady rhythm. Not noisily, right in your ear, but near to you, perhaps as you lean into them while they are holding or supporting you. Being held by someone who is breathing calmly and deeply can be very soothing in its own right (it is one tried and tested technique for calming babies who cry inconsolably for their first weeks of life) as well as helping you to re-establish your own breathing pattern once more.

Having a partner alongside, breathing in the right rhythm, is particularly important for women who have had pethidine, as the drug can occasionally cause them to become so relaxed that they forget to breathe at all.

MENTAL RELAXATION

Now that your body is relaxed, it is time to still your mind.

Sometimes when the body relaxes the mind goes into overdrive, imagining detailed conversations with people you know, having creative ideas relating to work, making shopping lists – anything rather than allowing you to switch it off for a while. However, you can often soothe, still and focus your mind by visualization, which means imagining something so clearly that you can see it in your mind's eye.

During the seventeenth century in France, women in labour often had a lighted candle and a particular type of rose, the Rose of Jericho, in holy water placed next to them. The heat of the burning candle made the rose's petals open out gradually, mirroring the way her body was slowly opening to let her baby out. This particular rose also had a special religious meaning as it was said to have blossomed for the first time at the birth of Christ, closed when he was crucified, and then opened again the day he rose from the dead (its other traditional name was the Resurrection Flower).

Just as the French women of 300 years ago concentrated on a real rose opening and imagined their bodies doing the same, today women are often taught in relaxation for childbirth classes to visualize their cervixes opening up like flowers unfolding. For many women, though there isn't a real flower to fix on, the visualization has a similar effect to watching one, in that this too can encourage their cervixes to dilate smoothly.

Other images which can be helpful and relaxing include a peaceful scene in the country, a deserted beach you once went to, a place under a tree by a river, a favourite armchair by the fire – anywhere where you feel secure and happy. Try to recreate all the details of how it looks, as if you are painting a picture of it in your mind, and hold it there. Soon you will be concentrating on that rather than on all the things you are supposed to be doing rather than relaxing (see also **Self-Hypnosis**, below).

It is far easier to do this when your body is relaxed and your breathing deep, than when you are in your usual state of consciousness.

Another way to use visualization in labour is to imagine any pain itself in a different way – perhaps seeing the contractions as huge, warm, rolling waves that you can float or ride over, flowing onto a peaceful, empty beach.

Visualize your body doing what it needs to do gently and well: perhaps your cervix softening like a ripe fruit, slowly opening up like the petals of a flower. See your baby moving steadily down the vagina, which you could visualize as soft and stretching easily.

When you feel rested and ready, wake yourself up gradually. Wriggle your fingers and toes, stretch, yawn, open your eyes, wait a few moments, then get up slowly.

Do not try to get up immediately as your blood pressure may drop measurably during deep relaxation and you could feel dizzy or faint if you scramble to your feet too fast.

WHEN CAN I USE THESE TECHNIQUES?

At any time you like. Especially helpful times include:

- When your contractions are starting to become regular and show a pattern, to help you ground yourself at the beginning of your labour.

- When they start to feel painful.

- At any time during the first stage. Imagining your cervix opening steadily and gently can be very helpful, especially if you appear to have become 'stuck' at a certain dilation point for a while.

- During transition. If you try to shut out everything else for a while you can imagine yourself in a calm place where only you are allowed to set foot.

- If the contractions are becoming very frequent and intense and you feel you are losing your ability to cope with them try visualizing them as waves and see yourself riding them or floating with them (see above).
- As you are pushing your baby out, visualize your birth canal as soft and stretchy.
- After your baby's birth.

Some women report that deep breathing and relaxation was helpful when they had the blues on the third or fourth day after their baby was born. Others say they visualized lots of milk coming through into, and streaming out of, their breasts and that this helped them establish breastfeeding. Deep relaxation and slow breathing are also useful for helping you getting to sleep – or back to sleep – at night, both in a rather noisy hospital maternity ward and when you bring your baby home.

WHEN CAN'T I USE THESE TECHNIQUES?

No known contraindications. Can also be used with all forms of pain-relieving drugs.

HOW QUICKLY DOES IT WORK?

Can have a calming effect within a few minutes.

HOW LONG DOES IT LAST?

Throughout labour; and can leave you feeling calmer afterwards, even when you have stopped using the technique.

Pros

- Can offer good pain relief.
- Under your own control.
- No adverse side effects for you or your baby.

- Can use it at any point during labour, and useful afterwards too.

- No circumstances under which it would not be helpful.

- Can combine it with all other forms of pain relief if required.

Cons

- Takes time and practice to learn. You would, for best results, need at least a month of antenatal classes and home practice to become sufficiently used to doing it, for it to be of real help during labour.

- There will be a fee for NCT and Active Birth classes ranging from £30 to £90 (depending on which area you live in) for an eight-week course of two-hour classes. Hospital antenatal classes will probably tell you about the technique, but will not have much time to devote to showing you how to do it – perhaps a single lesson to give you the basic idea.

- Does not offer total pain relief.

- Does not work well for all women, as some find relaxation techniques much more difficult than others.

HOW DO I GET IT?

See **Resources** for details of organizations which run classes.

ACUPUNCTURE

WHAT IS IT?

An ancient Chinese form of medicine involving the insertion of fine needles into different parts of the body to treat illness and soothe pain. It is still widely practised in China today, and is rapidly gaining acceptance in Western societies as well, especially in the field of chronic pain relief.

HOW DOES IT WORK?

Acupuncturists trained in the traditional Chinese techniques work on the principle that there are hundreds of small points scattered all over the skin's surface, which are linked to particular organs or functions of the body, by invisible energy paths called meridians.

Energy, which the Chinese call Chi and which some Western scientists have suggested exist in the form of electromagnetic energy, travels constantly and steadily round the body along the meridian pathways, like electricity flowing around a delicate, complex circuitboard. According to research conducted by scientists at the Institute of Electrical and Electronic Engineers the areas of skin above the meridian paths do show specific electrical properties which the skin on either side of the said paths does not have.

Practitioners of acupuncture believe that illness or disease is caused when this moving energy becomes blocked in a particular meridian or organ, causing a disruption or starvation of energy in the area it usually supplies. They deal with this by using fine needles inserted into the troubled acupressure points concerned to unblock the energy flow and get it moving smoothly again.

In addition to relieving pain, acupuncture can also be used to stimulate strong womb contractions and encourage an overdue labour to begin.* There have even been documented cases of it turning breech births† and of its use as the only form of pain relief for a caesarean section.‡

Acupuncture is now used in several British NHS pain clinics to give respite from chronic problems ranging from impacted spinal discs to intractable arthritis.

---

* *The American Journal of Chinese Medicine* 1976.
† The Shanghai College of Traditional Medicine's *Acupuncture – A Comprehensive Text*, 1984.
‡ *The Chinese Medical Journal*, 1980.

HOW DO YOU USE ACUPUNCTURE?

An acupuncturist would stimulate certain points, usually in the ear and sometimes on the hands and feet using hair-fine sterilized steel needles about the length of a long dressmaking pin. They look as if they ought to hurt when put in, but usually you will barely feel them being inserted. Some women do not feel the needles at all, others report a tingling sensation as they are used.

Usually the therapist will move the needle slightly to produce what is called a needle sensation (felt as warmth, or a mild electrical tingle). Then they will stop stimulating that needle and simply leave it in place to do its work.

To provide pain relief in labour needles are usually placed in the feet. If, however, the woman prefers to be able to move around freely, her acupuncturist would place the needles in the points in her ears or even her hands.

You would usually have between two and five needles inserted, which may either be left in for about half an hour, or removed after only a few minutes and reinserted during the later part of the first stage of labour. They may be left still, or the therapist might occasionally turn or move them very gently.

There is another type of acupuncture, called electro-acupuncture, which is often used for women in labour. To give the area extra stimulus, the therapist would use needles wired up to a gentle source of electricity. Whilst plain needles are left in for 10 to 20 minutes, electro-wired needles are left in place for longer. This is especially popular with Western acupuncturists and orthodox doctors who have had some acupuncture training.

Other variations include acupressure, which uses fingertip pressure – or even the points of elbows and knees – to stimulate the pain-relieving points. This is also known as *shiatsu*.

During the early part of labour a herb called Moxa may be used. This is bound into small bundles and lit so its aromatic smoke warms an area of skin around certain pressure points.

HOW EFFECTIVE IS IT?

Acupuncture can be so effective that in China, it is often used as a total block anaesthesia for caesarean sections instead of epidurals or general anaesthesia. For instance, between 1966 and 1985 doctors at the Beijing (Peking) Gynaecological and Obstetric Hospital, where 7,000 babies are born every year, carried out 5,000 caesareans using acupuncture alone. They are continuing to do so at the rate of 1,000 more every year.

Several published clinical studies have tried to assess just how acupuncture reduces pain. Findings include two possible explanations:

1. There is a hormone called serotonin which plays a significant part in labour by stimulating your womb to contract, and helping to create an awareness of pain. One Russian study found that acupuncture helped reduce or normalize serotonin levels.

2. The stimulation of certain pressure points releases some of the body's natural painkillers, which reduces the severity of pain during delivery.

For ordinary labours it is used to reduce pain rather than deaden all sensation. How far it can reduce pain without producing total numbness varies from woman to woman, and it suits some better than others. A small proportion of mothers will experience a virtually pain-free labour; others will find it of little help.

A study of two groups of 85 women at the Queen Mother's Hospital in Yorkhill, Glasgow* suggested that women who had the acupuncture felt calmer and more in control of their labours. The report concluded that from a pain relief point of view, the therapy had 'a significant part to play in the control of labour pain'.

As to how many women find it helpful, a study in the medical journal *Anaesthesia & Analgesia* in 1975 suggested that about two thirds of women do. In two other studies reported in the

* Published in the *Midwives Chronicle* in 1988.

late 1970s* between 60 and 90 per cent of first-time mothers and 90 per cent of mothers who had had babies before said acupuncture had given them 'significant' pain relief. According to the organization Acupuncture for Childbirth, on average it reduces pain for normal births by an estimated quarter to a third – taking a substantial edge off the pain rather than killing it altogether.

It can also help to strengthen contractions so that a slow, exhausting, apparently non-progressing labour goes more efficiently.

WHEN CAN I USE ACUPUNCTURE?

At any point in the first stage of labour once it has become established, but not for the second pushing and delivery stage when the midwives or doctors will become more involved – the acupuncturist usually retreats at this point. Acupuncture can also help with many of the problems you may have a few days after the birth: to promote breastfeeding, or encourage the healing of any stretches, cuts or tears, and help the womb return to its normal size.

WHEN CAN'T I USE ACUPUNCTURE?

There are no documented contraindications, in other words no particular type of person or particular instance which would mean acupuncture could not be used. It can also be used with other forms of pain relief – with one exception: electro-acupuncture cannot be used to provide pain relief in baths, showers, pools. Discuss with your acupuncturist also if you are considering using TENS at the same time.

HOW QUICKLY DOES IT WORK?

It can take effect within an hour or so.

* 'Acupuncture anaesthesia in normal delivery', *American Journal of Chinese Medicine*, 1977 and a report presented at the International Conference on Acupuncture in Sri Lanka in 1978.

HOW LONG DOES IT LAST?

For between 30 and 60 minutes after treatment, but some beneficial aftermath may continue for up to 24 hours later.

Pros

- Can be very effective; at the least it is said to usually take a substantial edge off any pain.

- Does not involve the use of drugs.

- The needles only go in a small way and do not hurt. If they do, say so immediately as they are not supposed to.

- No documented after-effects on the mother or her baby.

- You can usually remain mobile with acupuncture needles in, as long as they are in the ear area. If you need the stronger simulation of electro-acupuncture you would need to stay in one place but could still change positions, to lean over a beanbag or chair, squat, stand, etc.

- Can be used to help labour go smoothly in other ways too. However, if you would like to use acupuncture as anything other than a pain relief method, discuss this first with your midwife/obstetrician. It is best to include it in your birthplan (see pp. 7–10) or to raise it at one of your antenatal appointments, so if there are any problems you can sort them out then.

- A few prior visits to the acupuncturist(s) should get you in good condition for labour and recovery afterwards.

Cons

- Time-consuming preparation, preferably involving *at least* two or three sessions with your acupuncturist(s) beforehand.

- If your acupuncturist is using electro-acupuncture, this means additional wires and machinery. The equipment will also have to be switched off during fetal monitoring.

- Pain relief can be very variable.

- Can prove costly: fees are roughly between £15 and £30 for each prepartory session, after a first long initial consultation which would cost more. Then there is the fee for attending your delivery on top of that.

• You may have difficulty getting a hospital to agree to having your acupuncturist with you in labour.

It means having an extra person in your small room or cubicle for a large part of the time. You may feel crowded if your partner, a midwife (for intervals at least), your acupuncturist and occasionally a doctor are all in there with you.

HOW DO I GET IT?

First of all you need a professionally trained acupuncturist who has a special interest in pregnancy and childbirth. If you contact the Council of Acupuncture in London (see **Resources**) they should be able to tell you which of their members in your area can help.

Word of mouth is always an effective way to find good complementary practitioners of all types. Your local Active Birth group or NCT branch may know of someone, as may your community midwives or other mothers. Ring any contacts they give you and discuss what you would like over the phone first. Then, when you meet them, make sure you like and feel at ease with them. If you do not, no matter how experienced they seem to be, it would be best to find someone else.

Ideally you need to make contact with two, or even three such practitioners, as there is no guarantee otherwise that any particular one will be available to help when you go into labour – they may be in the middle of a busy day seeing several patients and be unable to get away.

It is important to work out a fee in advance. Some may charge by the hour, which could work out very expensive if your labour is a long one. Others may suggest a flat fee of anything between £100 to £200. Check that this will not be higher if you need their help at night or outside normal working hours.

Ideally, you should try to see the practitioner(s) of your choice regularly during pregnancy. This will mean being treated once a month, or once every two months if you are already in very good health, by one or other of them to encourage your system to remain balanced despite the changes of pregnancy, and to begin to tone up for labour. This also gives you the opportunity to get to know your practitioners. They may advise one visit a week during the last month of your pregnancy.

Ask them to suggest some points on your ear or feet which you can stimulate yourself with a match head or even the tip of your finger as an early form of acupressure to keep you going until they arrive.

AROMATHERAPY

WHAT IS IT?

The principal is similar to that of herbalism in that aromatherapy draws on the healing power of plants. But instead of using part or all of the plant, it just uses the potent, distinctive-smelling essence, known as the plant's essential oil.

Originally seen in Britain as a gentle extra something masseurs and beauticians added to their massage oil to help relax their clients, aromatherapy oils can also have very powerful healing properties. In France, for instance, some oils were used by Dr Jean Valnet in the Second World War to treat the appalling wounds received by frontline soldiers. As a result the French take aromatherapy very seriously and only their qualified doctors may use the oils to help diagnose and treat certain types of illness, prescribing them even for internal use.

Over the past ten years in the UK aromatherapy has quietly been gaining acceptance in some areas of orthodox medicine, and is now used with massage for premature babies, cardiac victims, cancer, people with AIDS, and in chronic pain clinics. Some of the small but growing number of new multi-disciplinary GP practices employ an aromatherapist once or twice a week with other complementary practitioners such as osteopaths, to work alongside the usual GPs and practice nurses.

HOW DOES IT WORK?

It is thought that the essential oils act as triggers on areas of the central nervous system, producing a measure of pain relief by stimulating the release of certain neurochemicals including the naturally painkilling endorphin group.

Different essences are said to stimulate the release of different types of neurochemicals. Some are thought to work by encouraging the output of your body's own sedative, stimulant and relaxing substances. Many also appear to be anti-infective, killing viruses, bacteria and fungal infections, which means they can also be very helpful after delivery if you have any problems such as infected stitches.

There are more than 200 essential oils in all, though only 30 or 40 which are commonly used, including cedarwood, lemon, rosemary, rose, lavender, ginger, myrrh, cypress, and juniper berry. A single oil may have more than one property.

HOW EFFECTIVE IS IT?

Aromatherapy has been successfully used as a method of pain relief in labour at several maternity units, including those in Ipswich and Southampton. It has also been studied by the midwives at Oxford's John Radcliffe Hospital: their results were published in the *Nursing Times* (March 1994). The oils were given to 585 women in labour as pain relief, to calm, to reduce nausea, and to increase the rate or strength of the labour contractions: 62 per cent said the oils were effective for them, 12 per cent said they did not help (the rest were not sure).

The scientific research committee of Britain's umbrella body for professional aromatherapists, the Aromatherapy Organizations Council, is currently doing a study of 1,000 women whose midwives or aromatherapists used essential oils to help soothe their pain during labour. Their initial results suggest beneficial effects.

According to the AOC's Director of Scientific Research, former pathologist Dr Vivienne Lunny who trains midwives and nurses in the use of essential oils, the pain relief the oils cans offer is variable. Still she says that most women would rate its effectiveness at 'between 60 and 70 per cent. This could be even higher – up to 85 per cent – if you had a trained therapist, or a midwife who was trained properly in the use of oils.' Aromatherapy is now becoming increasingly popular amongst midwives, even including the very senior professionals, such as Margaret Mason who is the tutor in Midwifery Studies at Southampton General Hospital.

HOW DO YOU USE AROMATHERAPY?

There are several different ways to use aromatherapy oils.

1. Breathe them in

You can either inhale them in a steam infusion by bending your head over a basin of very hot water or holding a beauty-mask steamer to your face, or by applying a few drops of neat oil to a cloth such as a cool damp face flannel and holding it up to your nose. Other ways of administering them include putting a few drops on a piece of absorbent card for inhaling, or putting drops on a pillow or beanbag you are using.

According to the Midwifery team at Oxford's John Radcliffe Hospital, peppermint can be put as a droplet on your forehead – though some women complained that this stung – and frankincense may be given as a droplet on the palm of your hand.

When you breathe them in, the essential oil particles come into immediate contact with the roof of both nasal passages. There are tiny sensory cell receptors buried in the protective mucus lining of these passages, and protruding from each one, thin hairs called cilia which register and transmit information about the smell you have just inhaled via the olfactory bulb at their root.

From here, electro-chemical messages race to the limbic area of the brain, which is associated with your sense of smell. This is thought to trigger the release of a variety of different neurochemicals. If you have just inhaled an essential oil with sedative properties like cedarwood, for instance, aromatherapists feel this encourages your brain to release neurochemicals to make you calm and slightly drowsy. Lavender, which can, amongst other things, help soothe pain, is thought to trigger the release of neuro-chemicals from the endorphin group. These are morphine-like substances, some of which act as natural analgesics. They are produced in impressively large quantities by your body when you go into labour, and are also involved in several other natural pain-relieving methods, notably water, TENS, acupuncture and reflexology.

Most of the oils have more than one type of action. It is not unusual to find one which is said to have analgesic properties but which can also induce drowsiness and promote sleep (certain painkilling drugs such as morphine and pethidine have the same effect). Lavender oil is one example of this. The John Radcliffe Hospital midwives survey found it helped reduce labour pain, and research published in July 1994 in the *Nursing Times* reported that a drop of this oil placed on the pillow at night could improve the quality of sleep for elderly people.

2. Mix the essential oils with a carrier oil and massage them onto the skin

Massage alone can help reduce pain in labour (see pp. 188–98), but aromatherapists and many midwives say it is far more effective if you use essential oils as well.

Generally the skin is an efficient barrier. However, very small amounts of essential oil have been shown to seep deep into the pores and hair follicles. Because these structures are rooted in the lowest, living layer of skin, just above the network of blood vessels and nerves this is thought to be the route by which the oils reach the blood capillaries.

Once they get there they can be transported around the body, and if even tiny amounts reach the nerves, they have direct access to the central nervous system itself.

In the first stage of labour, try a lower back massage with a carrier oil containing a blend of lavender, melissa, clary sage, jasmine and rose. Applied for 10 to 15 minutes every half hour, this can help relax your muscles and raise your pain threshold.

On the second stage, you can do lower back, foot, face, scalp, neck or shoulder massage with the same oils for as long as the woman wishes, to help with the pain of contractions.

NOTE: Some women simply do not want to be touched much when they are in labour so being massaged or being asked to inhale essential oils might irritate and upset them. Instead, they may find a bath containing essential oils more comforting. Or you could try putting several drops of lavender and clary sage on the neckline of their gown or T-shirt, on their pillow, beanbag, or even their front hairline if they like the smell.

3. Add several drops of essential oil to a bath

Again, small quantities of the oil will be absorbed via your hair follicles and skin pores, and some will be breathed in through water droplets of steam in the air.

Do not make the bath too hot. It could make you dizzy and it can also raise the baby's temperature. You need to stay in the water for at least 20 minutes to get the full effect.

Lying or sitting in a bath of warm water can be very helpful in itself for soothing pain in labour (see pp. 178–88) with or without oils. But it is also a good way to use essential oils – add between 6 and 10 drops (but check with your midwife first). A study of around 600 women carried out by midwives at Oxford's John Radcliffe Hospital in 1993 showed that when lavender oil was added to the water, the women felt considerably less pain and had far shorter labours than those who used baths without any essential oils added.

Helpful oils for pain relief
- Lavender (must be the *Lavendula angustifolia* variety, check with the supplier as there are several varieties of Lavender and not all are analgesic). This has an analgesic and slightly sedative, calming effect.
- Clary sage.

- Camomile

Oils with a calming or uplifting effect

- Frankincense
- Melissa
- Rose (this may be too overpowering a smell for some women – or too expensive, see below)
- Rosewood
- Neroli
- Jasmine
- Bergamot
- Lemon
- Mandarin

If the woman in labour does not like the smell of one of the oils, do not use it. Find an alternative instead. Many women are especially sensitive to smell when they are giving birth to a baby, and no matter how helpful it may be physiologically, it is going to do more harm than good if the scent itself is distressing her.

WHEN CAN I USE AROMATHERAPY?

At any stage of your labour, right from the earliest few contractions. The aromatherapy oils advised for use in labour do not interfere with the way the womb works.

WHEN CAN'T I USE AROMATHERAPY?

Do not use oils when pregnant or in labour without having consulted a properly trained aromatherapist first. Some can be harmful in pregnancy and childbirth (see p. 151).

HOW QUICKLY DOES IT WORK?

Massage with essential oils or soaking in a warm bath to which the oils have been added, starts to take effect after about 10 minutes. You should feel the full effect after between 20 and 30 minutes.

If you are inhaling them, it takes only 2 or 3 minutes. The transport of the oils' messages to the brain is rapid, because they go via the olfactory nerves and the network of thin-walled blood capillaries in the nose, which are situated very close to the skin surface.

HOW LONG DOES IT LAST?

Each application probably lasts about 30 minutes to an hour, but this is difficult to judge as the massage can continue all the way through labour if the woman wishes.

Pros

- No negative effects on mother or baby have been recorded. This may be because there are none, but it may also be because little research has been carried out into the subject.

- Aromatherapy is compatible with other forms of pain relief, including drugs.

- Non-invasive.

- Can be most effective.

- Smells good, and so may be a welcome change from the usual smells of a hospital. May also be agreeable and calming to the other people present at the birth including the baby, your partner and midwife.

- Methods of giving aromatherapy are very soothing and pleasant in themselves, especially massage and warm baths.

- Can be very helpful after delivery too.

Cons

- The cost – though there are many ways of reducing this (see below). Aromatherapy in labour is not free on the NHS (unless you happen to be part of a clinical midwifery trial), and some of the oils can be expensive.
- The difficulty of finding a *properly qualified* aromatherapist who has a special interest in childbirth, and for who may be happy to come with you to hospital.
- A hospital may raise some objections if you wish to take your aromatherapist into the labour ward with you. This might require some tact, persistence and shopping around to resolve.

HOW DO I GET IT?

To find a professionally qualified therapist, contact the Aromatherapy Organizations Council (see **Resources**) and ask which of their members has an interest in helping women in childbirth. It is very important to have the help of an aromatherapist who has been properly trained and knows what they are doing if they are going to treat you in pregnancy or labour.

AOC members' fees are a little higher than for therapists who have not done any of the recognized training courses; the latter may only have had a very short course – sometimes no more than a weekend or two. This may be fine if they are offering basic relaxation massages and beauty treatments with essential oils, but they would not be qualified to help women in pregnancy or childbirth.

When you have some names and phone numbers of therapists, speak to them first over the phone, and explain to them what you would like. Aromatherapy for labour pain can be supplied in three ways:

1. An aromatherapist personally comes with you to the labour ward and stays with you until your baby has been born.

   A qualified therapist would probably charge a flat fee (negotiate it beforehand) of between £50 and £100. There would also be a fee of £20–£40 for an initial consultation with them, which would also include an aromatherapy treatment. Many will charge far less if you really need help and have little money, so if fees are a problem, talk this over with them first. Check that they are willing to come with you after-hours or during the night, as babies arrive at unpredictable times and they may have to spend all night with you then face a full quota of clients the next day.

Make sure that you like and feel comfortable with the therapist. If you don't, it's best to find someone else, no matter how good this one may be.

2. Use a pre-prepared birth kit of aromatherapy oils when you are in labour.

A cheaper option would be to go and see a therapist who has an interest in childbirth and explain that you do not need them with you in labour, but would like them to make up a birth kit for you of the most helpful oils. If you want to be massaged rather than putting the oils in a bath or on a flannel, also explain that you would like to show your partner (whether it is your husband, boyfriend, friend, mother, sister) the best way to massage you. This will cost between £20 and £40 for the consultation, and perhaps another few pounds for the mixture of oils (sometimes there will be no extra charge for this).

3. Phone consultation.

Least expensive of all, you can contact an aromatherapist who has an interest in childbirth and offer to pay for a phone consultation (between £5 and £10) for advice on which oils to use in your labour and in what quantities.

There are several good mail-order companies which supply professional therapists as well as members of the public. Their oils are usually of better quality than those sold in health shops or the budget varieties sold in franchises like Body Shop, which tend to smell good but be less effective. See **Resources** for addresses. Oils can be costly: lavender, clary sage and rosewood are £4 or £5 for a 10ml bottle (used together they may well provide helpful pain relief), but rose can cost from £25–30 for a mere 2ml, as can Jasmine and Neroli. Melissa is £20-plus for a 10ml bottle. You may need to tailor your mixture of oils to your budget.

Having bought the recommended oils, take the mixture in with you to hospital or at home if that's where you are having your baby. Either ask your midwife to help massage your back with it (if they have time) or ask your partner to do it for you. It is not very effective to try and massage yourself during labour. Though you can certainly reach your lower back, it is not the same at all. If you can't get anyone to massage you, ask for access to a warm bath – nearly all labour units have them – put 10 drops of oil mixture in it and have a long soak.

WARNING

- If you are pregnant, do not have treatments with an aromatherapist unless they have a proper professional training (contact the AOC).

- Treat aromatherapy with respect. The oils may appear to be nothing more than concentrated beautiful smells, but they can be very powerful, even downright harmful if used inappropriately. For instance there are some which may stimulate uterine contractions and cause miscarriage or premature labour.

- Beware of using cheap oils. They can cause skin rashes.

AUTOGENIC TRAINING (AT)

WHAT IS IT?

A deep relaxation therapy based on meditation through six simple mental exercises aimed at relieving stress.

There are said to be more than 3,000 published clinical papers giving details of its use to help with a variety of different health problems. It has been used medically in the UK, Europe, Russia,

Japan and North America to help with a range of clinical disorders including high blood pressure, asthma, colitis, irritable bowel syndrome, muscular pain, arthritis, migraine, PMS and bladder disorders. Many psychological problems benefit from AT too, especially anxiety, sleep difficulties and panic attacks.

AT has also been successfully used, in documented clinical trials, to reduce pain in labour and speed up both the first and second stages.

The method was originally developed in Berlin by a German neuro-psychiatrist called Dr Johannes Schultz, who noted that hypnosis had a beneficial effect on the health of many of his patients. This led him to devise a set of five relaxation exercises which could achieve similar results without the need for hypnosis.

HOW DOES IT WORK?

By helping you to relax deeply and rapidly. Meditation has been described in many ways – but it is basically being completely focused on enjoying total peace and quiet, able to ignore interruptions, relaxing completely. It does not involve actually 'doing' anything: rather the reverse, because for once you are happily doing nothing.

HOW EFFECTIVE IS IT?

Since the late 1950s, Professor Prill of Wurzburg University's Department of Obstetrics has carried out several studies (one of which involved more than 1,000 mothers) on AT for pregnant women in labour. Much of the work done with pregnant women today is based on his work. They include the following:

- A study of 142 women in labour, in which 102 of them said the pain relief AT gave them was either good or very good, 23 said it was moderately helpful and 17 found it of little or no use at all

- Another piece of research looking at 302 women who had received AT training during their pregnancies found that about 70 per cent said they had 'notable pain relief'. Work carried out in Kyoto, Japan in 1967 and in Italy in 1961 and 1966 found similar results.

● AT appears to shorten the length of labour by an average of one third for both first and subsequent babies.

HOW DO YOU LEARN AT FOR PAIN RELIEF IN LABOUR?

The technique is taught over an eight to ten week period, either in a group or one to one. You need to start learning AT early, preferably no later than your sixth month of pregnancy. It should be practised two or three times a day while you are learning how to do it. Even when you have completed the course, daily practice is still advisable. At the very least, you would need to practise it two or three times a week. The more you practise, the better you will be at it and the more effective it will be.

There are six basic exercises, plus a session of peaceful meditation at the end of each one which you can use purely for relaxation, or as an opportunity to do an affirmation. An affirmation is an instruction to the mind, such as 'My labour will not hurt', 'My labour will go easily and naturally' or, if you are having sleep problems for instance, 'I will allow myself to fall asleep easily and quickly tonight'. Affirmations can be slipped in when you have meditated peacefully for a little while as by then your mind is very receptive to them.

The phrase in brackets is repeated three times.

Exercise 1

Heaviness: feeling a heavy relaxation in your arms, legs, shoulders and neck.
    ('My arms and legs are heavy.')

Exercise 2

Warmth: concentrate on feeling warmth in your arms and legs.
    ('My arms and legs are heavy and warm.')

Exercise 3

You may need to leave this one out as it can cause discomfort for pregnant women whose circulatory system is already working far harder than usual due to a 50 per cent increase in the amount of blood in their bodies. Discuss with your AT instructor.

Heart rate: concentrate on your own heartbeat.

('My heartbeat is calm and regular.')

Exercise 4

Breathing: making you aware of your breath.

('It breathes me.' This sounds thoroughly ungrammatical but what it means is that your breathing mechanism is working independently on your behalf – your body is literally breathing for you or 'breathing you'.)

Exercise 5

Pregnant women are advised to avoid this one too as the abdomen already has a considerable increase in blood supply and circulation because of the placenta and the warming effect of this exercise could increase circulation even further, having an adverse effect on the placenta's blood supply. Check with your AT instructor.

Abdominal warmth: focusing on a feeling of warmth in your solar plexus.

('My solar plexus is warm.')

Exercise 6

The forehead: concentrates on a feeling of coolness along the forehead.

('My forehead is cool and clear.')

And finally, as a way of allowing some quiet, calm meditation time:

('I am at peace.')

WHEN CAN I USE AT?

At any stage of labour you like. It can also be very helpful after the birth of your baby for general relaxation, and in helping to deal with the fourth-day blues which most women experience to some degree. AT practitioners also say it may be used to help to establish breastfeeding – and to get off to sleep quickly and easily after your baby has woken you at night (which many mothers find becomes progressively more difficult).

WHEN CAN'T I USE AT?

There are no known contraindications. AT is compatible with other methods of pain relief, should you find you need additional help.

HOW QUICKLY DOES IT WORK?

To be able to relax deeply and rapidly you need to have practised AT, just as you need to have practised any other natural method you do for yourself such as self-hypnosis or breathing and relaxation, for at least three months beforehand. Once you are able to do this, you can use it in several different ways:

- Going through the mental exercise routine once, twice or three times to achieve and remain in a state of deep calm and relaxation throughout your labour.

- Do your full AT routine when your labour is beginning then add in an affirmation at the end, to the effect that your labour will be smooth, rapid and pain free.

- The most effective way to use AT in labour is thought to be to adapt the mental exercises and the passive concentration they produce to coincide with the rhythm of your labour pains, so that the deepest and most effective part of each exercise ('It breathes me', see above) coincides with the peak of each contraction.

If you are you doing the full routine from one to three times (the usual way of producing relaxation in ordinary circumstances) it would take between about 8 and 20 minutes to complete. The AT would begin to have some effect on your levels of relaxation and perception of pain straight away, with its fullest effect coming into force as soon as you have finished the exercises.

However, if you are doing these exercises repeatedly and timing them to coincide with your contractions, the full effect of AT's pain relief should occur at the same time as you are doing the routine.

HOW LONG DOES IT LAST?

The pain-relieving effect can last for as long as it is needed.

Pros

- Under your own control.

- Helpful to some extent for about three quarters of women.

- No adverse effects during or after use for either the mother or her baby.

- Helpful for other difficulties after the birth.

- Unlike other forms of deep relaxation and meditation such as yoga and transcendental meditation, it is possible to learn AT quickly and get appreciable results (such as more peaceful sleep) within as little as a week or two.

- Once learnt, it is an easy and effective method of stress reduction for all kinds of circumstances.

Cons

- It takes practice, and it can be difficult finding the time for this if you have other children at home needing your attention, or you are still working while pregnant – or both.

- Can be time-consuming going to eight weekly training sessions – especially if you are going to weekly antenatal classes as well.

- Costs money to take an AT training course: between £90

and £150 or so for a group course, and more for individual tuition.

- Does not offer total pain relief.
- Does not work for everybody.

HOW DO I GET IT?

You need to find a properly qualified instructor to teach you how to do AT. There are about a hundred qualified teachers countrywide. To find one in your area, contact the British Association for Autogenic Training (see **Resources**). A teacher will show you one exercise per week, and help you deal with any temporary difficulties which may arise from the training.

Some hospitals, such as the Royal London Homeopathic Hospital, have AT therapists on their staff, offering training and treatment on the NHS. However, these are generally reserved for medical and surgical cases: some are attached to cardiac units, for example, to help people who have had life-threatening heart problems.

WARNING

It is very important to have a teacher who also has proper qualifications in one of the caring professions, such as a nurse, doctor, counsellor or psychologist. AT can release long-buried psychological and physical problems which you may need temporary help to deal with should they come out. For the same reason, do not just use a book to teach yourself AT.

HOMEOPATHY

WHAT IS IT?

The word homeopathy is coined from an ancient Greek phrase meaning 'similar suffering'; that like will cure like. It is based upon three main principles:

- The ancient **Law of Similars**, which states that whatever can harm, can also cure that harm.
- The theory of **The Minimum Dose**, which means that to get a reaction you only need to use a tiny stimulus.
- The theory of **The Single Remedy**: that you should use only one type of remedy at a time.

HOW DOES IT WORK?

All homeopathic remedies work by gently stimulating the body's own defence systems so it can heal itself.

To help someone who is unwell or in pain, a homeopath would prescribe minute, safe doses of the things which can, in larger quantities, produce the very symptoms they are trying to cure. For women in labour, however, a homeopath chooses the right remedy according to which *type* or types of pain, *and* emotions, a woman says she is feeling.

These doses may be diluted tens of thousands of times, so diluted in fact that conventional methods of analysis can find no trace of the original substance left. But whereas with drugs the larger the dose, the more effective it can be, the opposite is true in homeopathy. The less of a homeopathic remedy you give someone, the more powerful its effect.

Coffea, derived from coffee, is one example. Several cups of coffee last thing at night can stimulate your nervous system and cause sleeplessness and jumpiness. But when the derivative is given in minute homeopathic preparations it has the opposite effect, soothing the nerves and promoting sleep.

This phenomenon was discovered by a German physicist and

chemist called Samuel Hahnemann in 1796. Disillusioned by the medical practices of his day – when doctors commonly used large doses of poisonous substances like mercury, or bled patients heavily (often killing them in the process) to 'draw off' their diseases – he gave up orthodox medicine.

Then one day he translated an English article about a type of Peruvian bark which could be used to cure malaria. He started experimenting with it, testing doses of the bark on himself, noticing that when he did so with tiny doses, he developed very mild symptoms of malaria – thirst, weakness, chilliness, and drowsiness. It was this that set him on the road to the discovery that minute quantities of a substance which can provoke certain symptoms may also help cure those same symptoms.

Examples of the more common remedies for labour pain, based on a woman's emotional state as well as the sort of pain she is having, include:

Arnica	to help reduce bruising, swelling and trauma. This is perhaps the best known and most widely used of all homeopathic remedies in childbirth; though a small study of 20 mothers in Sussex in 1994 said it made no difference to recovery.
Belladonna	for very violent, powerful contractions.
Bellis perennis	for any deep abdominal surgery, including caesareans.
Cimicifuga	for pains which shoot right across the front of your abdomen, or pains that go down your hips on either side. These may be irregular, and they may make you shiver and shake.
Coffea	if the pains are very strong and sore – often helpful for women who are usually highly active, and now experiencing excessively painful contractions.
Caulophyllum	needle-like pains in the cervix, which may leave a mother fretful and shivering. Also helpful for spasmodic, irregular and ineffectual contractions.
Gelsemium	for violent contractions which seem to be ineffective, and not dilating your cervix (which remains rigid).
Kali carb	for labours when all the pain seems to be in your

> lower back – especially if only very hard rubbing
> on it seems to give any relief.

And, for other forms of discomfort and distress:

Nux vomica	If you are continually wanting to pass water, and have a strong urge to push all the time before it is time to do so. Also for cramping, spasmodic contractions, especially if the mother is also very irritable.
Pulsatilla and Hypericum	For different types of emotional distress.

Remedies are used in combination with each other such as Arnica and Hypericum. Different remedies would be helpful at different points in your labour and delivery, and as your physical sensations and moods vary.

HOW EFFECTIVE IS IT?

It sounds as though something so subtle would be of little use in a powerful and often painful process like childbirth, but homeopaths say the reverse is true. They claim that many women need no conventional pain relief when their labours are being supported homeopathically.

There are anecdotal stories from midwives and doctors trained in homeopathy of breech babies turning into the right position for delivery, and caesarean sections avoided because of the correct use of these individually prepared remedies.

However, homeopathy does not reduce pain in the same way as a drug or acupuncture can. It will still be there, so this would not be the right therapy for someone who wishes for a totally painless childbirth.

What homeopathy does do is subtly stimulate a woman's own physiological processes so they function well and strongly. Rather than obliterate the sensations it helps her to cope with it and take it in her stride. It can also calm, soothe and relax her emotionally, which in itself can reduce the pain level substantially.

One advantage of homeopathy is that, because it merely stimulates your own natural responses and ability in childbirth, having used homeopathy does not detract from the sense of achievement in giving birth – which to many women is a very important consideration.

There are studies of homeopathic medicines used on women in labour, but most look at helping the birth to progress smoothly and swiftly. None that we could find looked specifically at pain relief in childbirth, though there are several other pieces of published research which suggest homeopathy is an effective form of analgesia for *other* types of severe pain, including that associated with tooth extraction, neuralgia and migraine. And several more studies suggest that homeopathy can be effective in dealing with other types of serious childbirth problems such as post-partum haemorrhage.

In one small study in 1990, the department of Obstetrics and Gynaecology at the University of Milan gave 22 first-time mothers Caulophyllum, and compared their progress with 34 other women in labour who received none. The homeopathically treated women had labours that were on average 90 minutes shorter than the other women's.

Another study in the same year at the Kiev Medical Institute tried giving homeopathic remedies to 102 pregnant women at risk of uterine problems during labour (including uterine inertia and post-partum haemorrhage). A further 104 women who had similar risks were given conventional medical treatment such as artificial oestrogenic hormones. Both groups received careful monitoring including scans, fetal cardiomonitoring and clinical examinations. The homeopathic treatments were found to be 'in our opinion at least as effective as traditional prophylaxis'.

In 1985 the Faculty of Odontology in Marseilles, France, did a trial on 60 patients with dental neuralgia to test the painkilling properties of Arnica and Hypericum, two of the homeopathic treatments commonly used for different types of pain in childbirth. In comparing the treatments to a placebo (dummy treatment) they found homeopathy was more effective. And in Italy, the Policlinic of Brogo Roma in Verona did a randomized double-blind controlled study of 60 migraine cases, again treating them with some of the remedies used for childbirth pain, including Belladonna. They found it reduced the percentage of migraines occurring in the treated group from 10 a month to 1.3 compared with the control group (who were on dummy medication) starting off by having 9.7 attacks a month and going down to 8.

Homeopaths often suggest women take Arnica Montana in labour to help reduce bruising and bleeding. In 1990 the Department of Obstetrics & Gynaecology, University of Witwatersrand, Johannesburg ran a trial involving 159 women who had just had an episiotomy or perineal tear which seemed to confirm this. However, the potency D6 was more effective than the D30 (the potency usually available over the counter in health shops).

HOW IS IT USED?

By taking the advice of a trained practitioner you could build up a small basic kit to take you through labour. But for the best results, remedies really need to be customized for you individually, and it is very helpful to consult a homeopath a couple of months before your baby is due. During your consultation, they would take everything about you into account, not only your age and previous medical history but your personality, temperament, what makes you feel better or worse, the foods you like or dislike, and even factors such as whether you like the sea or thunderstorms. This is because homeopaths believe that pain is inextricably linked with your emotions, because neurological pain impulses register in the part of the brain that is also responsible for emotion.

> Different mothers will express very different emotions in childbirth – no two will be exactly alike. So though there are some general remedies that will probably be helpful for most women in childbirth you have to treat each woman in labour very individually.
>
> *Bridget Cummins, a midwife and homeopath with her own practice in Ireland, who regularly attends women in labour and runs a mother and baby clinic.*

The remedies are available in:

Lactose tablets, about the size of a Haliborange vitamin C pill.
  You can suck these or crunch them.

Powder, or granule (like tiny ball-bearings) form. These can be
  dissolved on the tongue or given mixed into some water.

Liquid form, so you take it via a dropper on your tongue.

It is much easier for women in labour to swallow small drops of
liquid than continually crunch tiny pills, especially as sometimes
the remedies need to be taken every five minutes for short periods.
If you only have the pills, your partner or midwife can crush them
up in a plastic spoon and mix them with water so you can still
take them in liquid form.

  Its also worth knowing that some of the remedies can be used
for your partner too if they are getting worried or upset. Apart
from anything else, if they are distressed, it will also upset you
and distract you from what you are trying to do. Useful remedies
here are things like Aconite (to calm fear and worry).

  The remedies come in different potencies. Potency 6 is the
lowest, and it is this one that is usually available over the counter
in chemists. Potency 30 is higher, which you might also be able
to get from some specialist suppliers (see **Resources** for details).
High potencies – 200 and above – are very useful if a situation
is urgent and acute, but these are best prescribed by a trained
homeopath.

WHEN CAN I USE HOMEOPATHY?

Whenever you like, at any stage of the pregnancy, delivery or
after the birth.

WHEN CAN'T I USE HOMEOPATHY?

There are no known circumstances in which it would be inadvis-
able or dangerous to use it.

  It is not possible to overdose on homeopathy, and if it is the
wrong remedy it will simply have no effect at all.

HOW QUICKLY DOES IT WORK?

If the correct remedy is given in the right dose you get relief within a few minutes to half an hour at the most.

In an acute situation like labour, you can take a remedy every 5, 10 or 15 minutes as required, and when it starts making an improvement the dose is decreased. When the improvement is established you can stop taking it. If there is no improvement after three doses, it is the wrong one.

HOW LONG DOES IT LAST?

It varies, depending on which potency was used and how acute the situation is. If the dose is say a 200, you may only need to take it the once. If all you have available are potency 6 remedies, you may need to take them every 10 to 30 minutes.

Should it wear off, you can always have some more. It is not rationed or in set doses as drug pain relief is.

Pros

- Can be very effective in helping women cope with labour.

- Gentle and non-invasive.

- No recorded adverse effects for a mother or for her baby.

- Widely available – though you have to arrange it yourself.

- The medication itself is inexpensive if you are simply taking a homeopath's advice on general remedies for a birth kit.

- Can be used throughout pregnancy and labour, and can also help considerably with postnatal problems like sore episiotomy sites and breastfeeding difficulties.

- Can work quickly.

- Can be repeated as necessary.

- Can be used with other forms of pain relief.

- Though you have 'had' homeopathy to help you cope with the pain of childbirth, this in no way detracts from the fact that the achievement of giving birth is 100 per cent yours. For some women this is very important.

- The medical profession seems to find this one of the most acceptable of all the forms of complementary medicine, as there are five NHS homeopathic hospitals in Britain; and many stringent clinical trials documenting the therapy's use in different areas of medicine. This may be helpful if you wish to bring a homeopath into hospital with you.

Cons

- Will not offer pain relief in the conventional way.
- Cannot offer a painless birth.
- Effectiveness of homeopathy is reduced if other forms of pain relief are given too, especially if they are powerful analgesic drugs or strong complementary therapies like aromatherapy, because they literally sledgehammer its gentle effects.
- Can be expensive if you want a homeopath with you during the birth. Even if they do not attend the birth, you'll still have to pay for a professional's advice plus a birth kit of remedies.
- Though homeopathy is well accepted by many doctors – and many indeed are trained in it – not all hospitals, nor all consultants, are happy to let you have a homeopath with you in the labour ward (see pp. 125–6).

HOW DO I GET IT?

To find a homeopath who is also a medically qualified doctor, contact the British Homeopathic Association; the Hahnemann Society or the Society of Homeopaths will supply you with names of non-medically qualified homeopaths (who will have done three to four years' specialist training) in your area with an interest in pregnancy and childbirth.

If you want the homeopath to attend the birth, phone the practitioner and explain what you want before arranging an appointment to make quite sure this is something they could help you with. This is important, because not all therapists are willing to attend women in labour because of the uncertain hours. Attending a labour could well mean they have to be up all night, then see their usual quota of patients all the next day. (Remember to check with the hospital that there is no objection to your therapist attending the birth.) Make sure that you like and feel comfortable with the practitioner. If you do not, it would be best to find another qualified homeopath to attend the birth.

Fees may be a stumbling block. Charges for the initial, in-depth consultation vary countrywide, but the average is £30 to £50. Subsequent consultations during pregnancy to help prepare your body for labour and recovery afterwards will be shorter and will cost less. Remedies are usually included in the consultation fee. To attend an actual birth, they may suggest a flat fee of about £100, or they may charge by the hour. The latter can mean you end up with a far larger bill than you had imagined, as it is never certain how long a baby will take to arrive.

A less expensive option than having the homeopath actually attend the birth would be to ask them to prescribe some remedies to see you through your pregnancy and recovery, and to give you a personal birth kit for you and your partner to use on the day, along with a careful explanation of how to use it. Ask if, and how, it would be possible to contact them for any urgent advice after-hours, should you need it. This is worth checking; something unanticipated may come up during the labour which could be helped homeopathically, as long as you get the right advice.

You need not feel awkward about phoning your homeopath during labour if necessary. Some women's birth partners are in constant touch with the homeopath who is helping them by phone throughout labour, and as the practitioner has an interest in helping pregnant and labouring women he or she will be used to this. If you already have one (or can borrow one) a mobile phone is a great advantage here. If not, get your partner to take a large amount of change in case they need to make heavy use of the hospital pay phone.

If you can't afford a homeopath's fees, try reading up a little about how homeopathy works and draw up a small list of suggested remedies. Helpful books include *Homeopathic Medicine for Pregnancy and Childbirth* by Richard Moskowitz, MD (Natural Alternative Books, 1992) and *Alternative Maternity* by Nikki Wesson (Optima, 1989). Or ask for advice at a specialist homeopathic pharmacy (see **Resources**).

A typical birth kit might include: Bellis perennis in case of cuts (episiotomy and caesarean), Arnica to help reduce bleeding, Aconite to help calm fear in panic, Kali phos for exhaustion and feeling you cannot cope, and, for first-time births which not infrequently involve substantial labour pains which do not seem to be dilating the cervix, Gelsemium.

The remedies cost between £2 and £3 per bottle from suppliers, all of whom will send them to you by post. It would also be worth buying them in liquid or soft tablet form from the same suppliers.

If you are having a home birth, as 7,000 women do each year in Britain, check with the midwife or head of the midwifery team caring for you as to what their policy is on homeopathy. It is unlikely to be a problem because many midwives are now becoming interested in the benefits of homeopathy.

HYPNOTHERAPY

WHAT IS IT?

Hypnosis puts you into a very relaxed state of mind, similar to the way you feel when you are just about to fall asleep. But you are also:

- Very receptive to suggestion, providing it's not contrary to your moral, ethical or common sense code
- Able to concentrate intensely
- Able to edit out of your consciousness anything distracting or distressing, including pain.

Though hypnosis is often presented in stage shows and variety performances as something uncanny and magical, there is certainly nothing magical about it. Natural trance states occur all the time in everyday life. For instance, if you are trying to talk to someone who is immersed in a newspaper or TV programme, they may answer without even looking up at you, yet later deny ever having spoken at all. This is a good example of the human brain's ability to concentrate exclusively on one thing while choosing not to acknowledge or process any other incoming data. The effect is to programme the mind not to register any information it does not want to know about – including pain signals. Hypnosis is just a method of tuning the brain in to this extreme concentration mode.

Hypnosis will not:

- Send you to sleep, unless you are trying to actually get to sleep and using hypnotherapy as a means of doing so

- Make you do anything against your will or better judgement. The hypnotherapist merely gives you suggestions which you may follow or not as you wish. You do not give up control of your behaviour.

- Make you give any private secrets. Just as when you are awake, you decide what you are going to reveal and to whom. If hypnotherapy is used as part of psychoanalysis or counselling to help someone speak about a traumatic event or distressing time of their life, it merely makes it easier for the person to talk about what is troubling them. It will not make them do so against their will.

HOW DOES IT WORK?

What hypnosis can do is give you your own personal method of control over several physical functions within the body, from your heart and breathing rate to your perception of pain.

Pain perception: Hypnosis enables you to control the amount of pain you register far better than you could in your normal wide-awake state. It is also possible, with practice, to produce a numb feeling in any part of your body so successfully that operations have been perfumed under hypnosis rather than general anaesthetic. For instance, Dr Les Brann, a Chelmsford GP who has trained several hundred women to use hypnosis in their child-births, and works very closely with his local maternity unit at St John's Hospital in Chelmsford, cites the case of a caesarean performed there recently using only a very light epidural and hypnosis.

This is done by using a well established pain-control-through-hypnotherapy technique called glove hypnosis. The way it works is that the woman in labour concentrates on allowing one of her hands to become totally numb (they are often told to imagine they are plunging their hand into ice-cold water). It is then poss-ible, with practice, to use that hand to pass on numbness to other parts of the body just by touching the area.

The technique is often taught to pregnant women learning self-hypnosis so they can use it in their labours to numb their abdomens, thus reducing the pain they feel from their contrac-tions. They can also use it to reduce sensation in their vaginal canals when the baby is being pushed out, or around their peri-neum and labia if they need stitches afterwards.

Muscles: These can be relaxed or encouraged to work at peak efficiency under hypnosis. Both can be very helpful for women in labour, as during the first stage and pushing stage muscular tension tends to create more pain. Relaxation can ease this.

It is also useful in helping your womb muscles to work at maximum efficiency when you are trying to push your baby out. Dr Brann, who has completed Sheffield University's degree course in hypnotherapy, has also done a good deal of research and work in this area with his local hospitals. According to him, there are many reports from doctors and midwives who have seen hypno-therapy used in labour, suggesting that it can shorten the second stage considerably.

Hypnosis is currently used in several NHS pain control clinics for the constant and severe pain created by problems as diverse as shingles, inoperable back injury, arthritis and certain types of cancer.

HOW IS IT USED?

You can be hypnotized by a therapist or you can be taught, by a responsible professional hypnotherapist, to hypnotize yourself very effectively. This means that the hypnotherapist doesn't actually have to be with you to provide pain relief in labour.

It takes a while to learn how to hypnotize yourself, and you need to practise during your pregnancy as often as you would practise breathing techniques or different active positions for labour. Once you have learned the technique you can use it wherever and whenever you wish without help from a hypnotherapist. A woman in labour who has mastered the technique should find she can concentrate deeply on calm, relaxation and effectively ignore at least some of the pain of her contractions.

IMPORTANT

Let your midwife and obstetrician know you are using self-hypnosis, and that you would appreciate some encouragement with it – which most midwives would offer anyway – rather than risk being asked 'What on earth are you doing?' at the wrong moment. They would also need to check the progress of your labour very regularly, and be aware that successful self-hypnosis might very occasionally mask problems in labour.

HOW EFFECTIVE IS IT?

The rather sparse medical research there has been in this area since the 1950s seems to suggest that it is a useful method of pain relief for childbirth.

Just how much it helps depends on the woman herself, because the physical perception of pain varies so much from person to person. It may only take the edge off, or it may give her a virtually pain-free labour. However, it is estimated that self-hypnosis can generally reduce the pain by about a third.

One study at the Aberdare District Maternity Unit in Mid

Glamorgan, Wales (1993) found that when they used hypnotherapy taught over six sessions, three times as many first-time mothers were able to do without any ordinary pain relief at all as those first-timers who had had no such training.

This particular piece of research involved 126 first-time mothers using the self-hypnosis they had been taught vs 300 controls who had been given no training, plus a further 136 mothers who had had babies before with another 300 controls. The hypnotized first-timers also had much shorter labour times – as short as if for a second or third baby. And the difference between the labour times for first and subsequent babies is considerable: an average of nine hours compared with four to six hours.

Another small trial in 1986 at St George's Hospital in London studied the difference in labour between 29 women using hypnosis and 36 who did not. The results showed no less need for pain relief amongst women using hypnosis, but that they had a shorter first stage of labour and said that their labour had been a better experience for using hypnosis. A 1986 trial in Essex by Dr Les Brann with 96 women using self-hypnosis or breathing again found shorter first stages of labour and more satisfaction in general about their childbirth for the hypnotized mothers.

Another study carried out between 1984–9 in Aberdeen on 262 first-time/subsequent mothers found hypnosis did indeed reduce the need for pain relief – especially for first-time mothers. It also found the first stage of labour was shorter for first-timers.*

What is more, it seems to have a positive effect on the baby. A report from the Fourth European Congress of Hypnosis in Psychotherapy and Psychosomatic Medicine (which took place in Oxford in 1987) suggested that babies born to mothers who had been hypnotized during labour were less likely to die. Another in the *Journal of the American Medical Association* (1960) suggested the babies of such mothers had higher Apgar scores when they were born – which means they were more alert, with better

* M. W. Jenkins, *British Journal of Obstetrics and Gynaecology*, Vol. 100, pp. 221–6.

reflexes – than babies whose mothers had not used hypnosis in their labours.

NOTE: If you feel more pain than you are able to cope with and self-hypnosis is not giving you as much help as you need, ask for another form of analgesia too. Hypnosis is compatible with all pain-relief methods and there is no reason why you should have to use this alone.

WHEN CAN I USE HYPNOTHERAPY?

At any stage of your labour. It can also be helpful afterwards for breastfeeding problems, post-delivery pain, the third- or fourth-day blues, and helping you make the most of what sleep you are able to get with a new baby to care for.

> 'I used it all the way through and it was brilliant. But my concentration slipped when I was pushing Jenny out – it all got too much – and yes, then it did hurt, but only for a very short while. I would definitely use hypnosis again.'

WHEN CAN'T I USE HYPNOTHERAPY?

There are no contraindications.

HOW QUICKLY DOES IT WORK?

Variable, but generally within half-hour or so.

HOW LONG DOES IT LAST?

For the whole of your labour and delivery if necessary, though you can keep reinforcing it yourself throughout.

Pros

- Non-invasive.

- Does not involve taking any natural remedies or pharmaceutical drugs.

- No known negative side effects on mother or baby.

- Under your own control.

- Can be helpful during pregnancy as well as in labour, and its usefulness need not stop after delivery. May be used for years afterwards to aid sleep, relaxation, etc.

- May make your labour shorter.

- May make a labour *seem* shorter. Under hypnosis, most people's perception of passing time changes and usually more goes by than they realize. And an eight-hour labour which seems like a five-hour one may be no bad thing.

Cons

- Can be expensive to learn.

- Can be time-consuming to find someone to teach you – especially if you have to organize a group of pregnant women to bring the costs of tuition down.

- Is not helpful for everyone.

- Self-hypnosis may work so successfully that you feel little pain, and this may confuse a midwife or obstetrician who is looking after you in labour. They may think that because you do not seem to be in much discomfort you are in a far earlier stage of labour than is actually the case. It is therefore important to have your labour's progress checked very regularly – which means regular vaginal examinations, preferably hourly, to see just how far your cervix has dilated. These may be more comfortable if they can be carried out while you are lying on your side or standing with one leg raised on the seat of a chair rather than traditional uncomfortable positions where you lie on your back.

- It is theoretically possible that hypnosis could mask the fact that a labour is obstructed in some way, again because the woman does not seem to be in much discomfort. We could find no cases of this on record however. Always be sure to let your midwife and obstetrician know that you are using hypnotherapy so they can be aware that problems might not be immediately obvious.

> 'I did a couple of hypnotherapy classes with three other women from my antenatal group. But though I wanted to, I just could not bring myself to believe that something like this could really protect me from pain that bad. And it didn't. I got really worried when the contractions began to hurt so I had pethidine as well, and then could not remember my self-hypnosis routine anyway.'

HOW DO I GET IT?

First you need to find a suitable hypnotherapist to teach you self-hypnosis. Try contacting either the British Society of Medical and Dental Hypnosis, whose members are all qualified doctors and dentists, or the British Society of Experimental and Clinical Hypnosis, which is open to doctors, dentists, graduate psychologists, and sometimes other professionals such as midwives and nurses. (See **Resources** for a list of helpful telephone numbers.)

When you are given the names and telephone numbers of any of their members in your area who have an interest in hypnosis for childbirth, speak to them first over the phone. Explain what you would like them to do, check up on their fees and any other practical arrangements. Then when you meet face to face, see how comfortable you feel with them, and whether you actually like them. If they are going to teach you hypnotherapy this is just as important as how well qualified they are, as you will not be able to learn well with them unless you feel at ease.

Besides medically qualified hypnotherapists, there are also many lay practitioners – therapists who have no medical background. Their training may be very extensive, or it may amount to a single weekend's tuition or even a correspondence course. There are more than 60 colleges offering hypnotherapy diplomas and it is difficult to tell for sure which ones train therapists well and which do not. However, in 1991 Sheffield University became the first in the world to offer a post-graduate diploma course in hypnosis for doctors, dentists and psychologists. London University has now done the same.

Once you have found a professionally qualified therapist whom you like and trust, there are two ways to learn self-hypnosis:

1. One-to-one sessions, which could teach you the self-hypnosis methods within two to three sessions. A private session with a medically qualified practitioner can cost from at least £50 an hour, which works out at £100 or more for a two-hour session. If you need two or three of these longer sessions, that comes to around £300.

2. Group sessions, usually of between 6 and 12 other women. You would usually need about six sessions. A handful of GPs and hospital antenatal units with an interest in the field offer such classes. They may be free, or they may have a low flat fee attached.

   If there are no courses like this in your area, another option is to get together a group of women from your own antenatal class who are interested in this and arrange group sessions with a therapist, dividing the fee between you. This will keep the cost down.

Whichever way you are taught it is also helpful to have a tape made for you that you can go away and practise with at home. Some therapists who do individual tuition will customize one specially for you. There is also a general tape and book (see **Resources**) on the market designed for women who want to use hypnotherapy throughout their pregnancy, during labour – and afterwards, to help combat sleep problems and breastfeeding difficulties.

Your course sessions will last from an hour to two hours, and you will be taught not only self-hypnosis but relaxation methods and probably visualization techniques as well to make it more effective.

Physical relaxation methods often involve deliberately making each part of your body in turn become heavy, floppy, or warm, until you feel loose and relaxed all over.

Visualization is literally seeing in your mind's eye the things you want to happen taking place in order to encourage them to do so. Some of the most usual images women are told to imagine in their mind's eye include their cervixes opening gently like the petals of a flower unfolding, or their contractions becoming strong and steady like powerful waves rolling in on the shore. You may also be taught to use visualization to help yourself feel calm and secure. What you might do here is to just imagine yourself in a peaceful place which makes you feel safe and relaxed, perhaps a favourite deserted beach, or a much-loved armchair by an open fire.

The actual self-hypnosis part will involve a series of mental exercises designed to help put you in a deeply relaxed, receptive state. Once you are in it, you can 'tell' yourself things or give your mind instructions, programming it to help your body behave as you want – whether this is to feel calm, not to feel pain, or not to notice time passing.

It is also possible to give your mind post-hypnotic instructions of things it can help you to do without thinking when you come out of your relaxed state, perhaps to have a swift, easy birth or not to feel nervous.

WATER

WHAT IS IT?

In its broadest terms, it is the use of warm water to relieve pain in labour (see fig. 9). This preferably takes the form of immersion in a small, purpose-built pool (sometimes permanent, sometimes portable). If a pool of the correct size is not available, an ordinary warm bath is very useful. Even warm showers can help considerably.

Few obstetricians or midwives would argue with the fact that ordinary warm water has both a calming and a pain-relieving effect on women in labour. However using water as an analgesic and actually giving birth to your baby in water are different things.

Many water enthusiasts are strongly in favour that actually giving birth in water is a gentle, safe, natural way to introduce a baby into the world. At the specialist centres which have water pools, of all the women who use them about two thirds get out to deliver their babies and the other third prefer to stay in. There are countless anecdotal reports of the pleasure, satisfaction and security that water births can offer, and some women speak of the sensuality of labouring and giving birth in water too.

At the moment, many obstetricians and midwives are concerned about the safety of the baby if it is born under water. Out of several thousand successful water births, there have been a few cases of babies' deaths and there are scientific reviews of the subject going on at the time of writing. This chapter is simply about using water as a natural method of pain relief. If you would like to find out more about giving birth to a baby in water, please see **Resources** for details of organizations which can give you a great deal of information.

HOW DOES IT WORK?

Water can work in several different ways to reduce the amount of pain you feel:

- It offers you privacy, as you will either be in a bathroom in a bath or shower, or in a birthing room with a pool. Either way you will be somewhere quiet and secluded rather than on a noisy hospital ward with curtains pulled round the bed, or on a labour ward where you are aware of other women in labour and staff coming and going. Privacy can encourage relaxation, and this in itself can reduce pain.

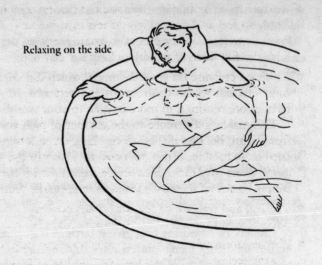

Relaxing on the side

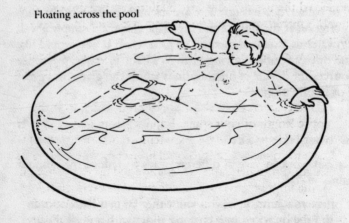

Floating across the pool

Immersion in warm water can help relieve labour pains. Many companies offer specially designed birthing pools for hire, and some hospitals have them on site. Ideally a birthing pool needs to be deep enough to immerse yourself in up to breast level when kneeling in it, and big enough for a second person to get in there with you if necessary.

- You are more mobile in water and can change positions easily. You also feel as if you weigh far less than before – a great contrast to how a very pregnant woman feels on dry land with the full force of gravity pulling her down.
- Lessened pressure on your abdomen, which can encourage more efficient womb contractions and better blood circulation, resulting in more oxygen to your womb muscles.

  This makes a difference to the amount of pain you feel from them, because if they do not have enough oxygen they become ischaemic. If this happens, they hurt in the same way as the heart may experience severe angina pain if the blood supply to any of its muscles is even temporarily reduced.
- The feel and warmth of the water can encourage you to relax physically and mentally, again reducing the pain you feel.
- The sensation of water all over your body can help to balance out the feelings of pain you are getting from one or two particular areas. Dr Yehudi Gordon, the obstetrician who pioneered the use of water for childbirth in Britain, says it is simply a matter of helping to even up the ratios of sensory impulses.

  Using water as a pain reliever is based on the Gate theory of pain put forward by two scientists called Wall and Melzack in 1965, which is as follows:

a) There is an area called the dorsal horn which runs the entire length of your spine. Impulses from nerves all over your body produced by pain, temperature or touch all have to connect with the dorsal horn somewhere along its length. From here, they are transmitted up to your brain.

b) Some impulses reaching the dorsal horn excite pain, others inhibit it. The amount of pain you feel depends on the balance between these different painful/painless impulses.

c) There are many different nerve fibres within the dorsal horn which transmit different types of stimuli at different speeds, pain impulses being transmitted more slowly than touch or pressure. Because touch and pressure sensations reach the brain faster than pain sensations, the former has the effect of damping down or muffling the latter before they can get to the brain to be registered as painful.

d) In this sense, they partially close the gate to pain sensations.

e) If you are getting plenty of pleasurable sensations coming in from all over your body because of the water's warmth and gentle pressure, this helps to block out pain you would otherwise be feeling. It is thought hat this is because it does not give many of those pain impulses the chance to travel up your spine and register with your brain. This holds true even though the pain impulses may be far more powerful than the pleasurable ones.

- Warm water encourages the secretion of endorphin hormones, which act as natural painkillers, mood uplifters and which may also have an oxytocic effect (ie can help stimulate strong womb contractions).

HOW EFFECTIVE IS IT?

Women react to pain in different ways and water cannot offer complete pain relief. What it can do is reduce the pain you feel to manageable levels – often so much so that you may not need additional methods of pain relief.

As water and natural childbirth pioneer Janet Balaskas describes it: 'Being in water does not take away pain as an epidural would, but it enhances your ability to cope with it by helping you relax very deeply. The pain remains challenging but it is easier to cope with it . . . you can experience the sensations at the peak of a contraction as intensity of feeling rather than pain, and are able to open up and go with it rather than resist it.'

WHEN CAN I USE WATER?

At any stage of your labour. According to Dr Gordon, women often find that if their labours have not been progressing well, things will start to improve once they have got into a warm pool or bath. Similarly, if labour is going very slowly or has stopped progressing for a woman who has been in the water the whole time, getting out can reverse the situation as being on dry land and being in water produce different atmospheres and states of consciousness. If a labouring woman changes her environment it can also produce a change in her labour progression – as many women who have been in full labour until the moment they arrive in hospital, whereupon everything stops, know to their cost.

Other natural methods of pain relief such as homeopathy, massage, self-hypnosis, yoga, breathing and relaxation, ear acupuncture (provided it is not the electro-acupuncture variety) or reflexology are all perfectly compatible with water.

Some midwives and doctors say there is no reason why you should not use Entonox while in water. If you want to do so, discuss this with your midwife, and perhaps try it and see how you get on. You would need a canister of the gas mounted on wheels rather than one attached to the wall, and should not be left alone in case you do suddenly feel dizzy or faint. TENS cannot be used if you are in water either, though it can if you get out after having been in a water pool as long as you are dried properly.

WHEN CAN'T I USE WATER?

During the first stage of labour water immersion is not advisable if:

• The baby needs continuous fetal heart monitoring. This is necessary where there are signs that the baby is in distress, such as meconium (the greenish waste which is the baby's first bowel movement) in the amniotic fluid when your waters break, or an abnormally rapid fetal heartbeat.
  There is one method of continuous monitoring which can

be used under water called telemetry, but this is not yet widely available. For intermittent monitoring, Oxford Sonicaid make a monitor suitable for use under water. Or you can get out of the pool temporarily, or even stand/squat leaning slightly forward over the pool's rim supported by your arms, so your abdomen is above the waterline for a while. This may be uncomfortable if the monitoring goes on for long.

- You are suffering severe pre-eclampsia with very high blood pressure, suggesting the possibility of full blown eclampsia. However, blood pressure tends to fall in water, possibly because it makes you more relaxed and calmer. But we do not know the effect on blood flow to the unborn child.

- If you have had any other form of pharmacological pain relief, like pethidine. Some doctors and midwives prefer you not to use water in case the drugs have made you unsteady on your legs, because there's a risk you may slip.

> You should you always have someone with you, regardless of whether you have had any pain-relieving drugs, if you are using a water pool during your childbirth.

HOW QUICKLY DOES IT WORK?

In about as long as it usually takes for a warm bath to relax you after a hard day. Full effects after 10–20 minutes.

HOW LONG DOES IT LAST?

For as long as you are in it. The calming effect may last for some time even after you leave the water.

Pros

Purely as a method of pain relief rather than an environment to also deliver your baby into, water's advantages include:

- A reduced rate of tears occurring in the perineum, vagina and

- Can help speed up a labour which does not seem to be progressing very well.
- Can reduce heightened blood pressure.
- The moist atmosphere in a room with a pool in it makes it easier to breathe (most maternity units have very dry and often overheated atmospheres). This can be especially helpful for women who have asthma.
- Ensures privacy. You cannot put a water pool, or even an ordinary bath, anywhere except in its own room.
- Warm water can be soothing and calming if you are feeling distressed.

'The water birth was brilliant. It made me very relaxed and therefore helped me to concentrate on my breathing.'

'I used a water tub in my own home and my baby was born at home. I have never had such a feeling of being so in control of something so powerful, and so calm and happy. I felt over the moon – I had done it all myself, my own way, and now I had this wonderful baby. I never got upset on the fourth day afterwards at home, like I did in hospital the previous time.'

'Having spent a fair bit of money on a hired pool, then with some difficulty persuaded the hospital to let me bring it in – I found I was perfectly comfortable with one of the bean bags they had there and being massaged; didn't want to move from it. I never even got into the water . . .'

Cons

- You may have some difficulty finding a hospital which either has a water pool or will let you bring in your own.

- If you use your own pool either at home or in hospital, you need to pay for it. See **Resources** under Active Birth Centre and Splashdown for information on costs.

- It is not recommended that a woman uses pain-relieving drugs which may cause dizziness or make her unsteady on her feet, and you cannot use a TENS machine either.

- A midwife who is unfamiliar with water immersion may worry about hurting her back bending over to look after you in a pool. There are special lifting/supporting techniques and recommended positions for those assisting women in birth pools: see **Resources** for where to find practical advice.

- Difficulty in monitoring the baby. Intermittent monitoring is not a problem, but continuous monitoring requires a waterproof battery-operated fetal monitor (see above: **When can't I use water?**)

- Faeces in the water: most women move their bowels to some extent during labour because the baby's head compresses the lower bowel tract, pushing out some of the waste matter inside it. If this happens while you are in a pool, it will end up in the water with you. Reports of water use do not show that this is a problem: if a bowel motion is passed it can be removed straight away with a domestic sieve kept next to the pool for this purpose. If the idea of faeces in the water upsets you, it may be useful to ask for a suppository during the early part of labour to help you empty your bowels. However, it is possible that this could make the problem worse, as any faecal matter remaining would be fairly loose and runny, and so more difficult to remove from the pool.

- Examinations can be more difficult. If the woman is kneeling or squatting in the water, this can make a vaginal examination rather awkward. The midwife would need to bend over the pool and put her hand and arm under the water as far as her shoulder to feel how far the cervix has dilated. However, it is no problem if the woman lies floating back against the rim of the pool. Checks on your temperature and pulse can be done regularly throughout labour without difficulty: a thermometer can be used in the usual way, and your blood pressure checked if you stand up out of the water.

HOW DO I GET A WATER POOL?

At the time of writing (autumn 1994) there are about 80 NHS and private maternity units offering a room with a birthing pool in the UK and by the time this book is published there will probably be even more.

There are also other centres which are happy to provide a room into which you can bring your own portable pool. These pools can be rented from two or three different companies from £100–£150 for 4 weeks (see **Resources**). To find out if any hospitals in your area offer their own birthing pool, contact the Active Birth Centre (see **Resources**). If you are having a home birth, again you can hire a pool for your own use there.

Most up-to-date obstetricians are happy for women to use water in general as a method of pain relief in their labours. Fewer are receptive to the idea of using it in the form of an actual birthing pool because of the space it takes up. They may suggest you use one of the labour unit's baths or showers instead.

However, while ordinary baths will certainly provide warm water they lack two of the most helpful characteristics of a proper birth pool: enough room for manoeuvre, and enough depth for buoyancy. Warm showers may provide warm water – but it can only be applied to one area of your body at a time unless you stand directly underneath it, and again it cannot offer the buoyancy and total relaxation of a pool.

If your hospital is not prepared to allow you to bring in a water pool, and you prefer not to use one of their baths as a substitute, try writing directly to the hospital's Director of Midwifery Services. If they are not receptive, write to the Unit General Manager and ask for his or her help, as they are often sympathetic. If you still have no luck (perhaps engineers and other technical staff need to be consulted about safety and general technicalities) your options for finding a hospital more kindly disposed to the idea include:

- Contacting your local Community Health Council (under C in the phone book) to see which units in your area would be amenable to it. CHCs collate information on all aspects of healthcare locally including maternity facilities, so they ought to have this information.

- Contact the Active Birth Centre, which has an up-to-date list of hospitals with pools.

- Ask your local midwives if they know of anywhere.

- Try the Royal College of Midwives, who have a good deal of information about midwifery practices countrywide.

- Ring one of the campaigning childbirth organizations such as AIMS or the NCT, who may be able to advise you.

MASSAGE

WHAT IS IT?

Essentially, massage is therapeutic touch which manipulates the body's soft tissues, which are the muscles, tendons and ligaments.

It is probably the oldest therapy known to humankind, having been used in the Far and Middle East since 3000 BC. Massage was very popular in ancient Greece – Hippocrates wrote in the fifth century: 'The way to health is to have a scented bath and an oiled massage every day.' The word itself probably comes from the Greek word *masein* meaning to knead, or from the Arabic word *mas'h*, which means to press softly.

In the language of the Navajo people of southwestern America, the woman who helps the mother give birth is The One Who Holds. This name for the birth assistant also describes the traditional idea of their main duties during the birth: to provide physical support for the mother – and to massage her. People massage women in childbirth nearly everywhere in the traditional world, except those where it is the custom for the mother to give birth alone.

The commonest ways to use massage are:

- to soothe and calm someone
- to help loosen and relax tense muscles.

Many complementary therapists such aromatherapists and osteopaths use massage as a standard part of their treatments. Reflexologists and shiatsu practitioners always use a form of specific modified touch and pressure for their work too.

Massage is probably most often used to help reduce stress, closely followed by certain types of circulatory problems such as high blood pressure, some forms of heart disease, certain sports injuries, occupational strains (perhaps from sitting hunched over a desk or driving wheel for hours) and psychological disorders including anxiety, addiction and depression. Most midwives, if they have time, automatically rub and massage women's backs during labour – and have probably done so for thousands of years. The trouble is that many maternity units are now so short-staffed that they often do not have the time.

'It was a loving touch when I needed it. I have always enjoyed massage and this was the one time in my life when I had a cast-iron excuse to have it for hours.'

'To my surprise, I found it got on my nerves – so I slapped his hands away (I think I was beyond speech by that time).'

'Just what I wanted.'
'Massage appeared to be helpful. But this might just have been the placebo effect in an attempt to convince me that my presence was not entirely useless . . .' *(a partner's view)*

HOW DOES IT WORK?

When it is used for women in labour, massage works in five different ways:

1. By restoring blood flow to stressed or damaged tissue: Muscles hurt during any prolonged major physical effort, including labour, because:

- The flow of oxygenated blood to feed the muscle fibres is interrupted. This happens because contracting muscles squeeze the blood vessels running through them and so restrict their own arterial supply of oxygenated blood into the area or the venous drainage routes leading out of it. Starved of oxygen (ischaemic), the muscles go into painful spasms.

  No one is entirely sure why muscles should hurt when their blood flow is restricted. One theory is that muscular activity generates large amounts of waste products, such as lactic acid, which are allowed to accumulate when the blood flow is interrupted. It has also been suggested that other chemical agents such as bradykinin and histamine are formed in the tissues because of muscle cell damage, and that it is these rather than the lactic acid which irritate and stimulate nerve endings in the muscle fibre, sensations which are experienced as pain.

- Muscular contraction speeds up the rate of metabolism of the tissues around it, which accelerates the onset of pain.

Massage is able to help relieve pain caused by the lack of oxygenated blood and the hyped-up metabolic rate of the surrounding tissues because the pressure of a deep kneading, or the stroking motion along the length of the muscle fibres, pushes fluid along in front of it. This encourages drainage of lymph fluid and of the deoxygenated blood carrying painful waste products from those muscles. It also encourages fresh oxygenated blood to flow in and replace the 'used and toxic' blood that is now on its way to the kidneys and liver for purification.

2. By combating muscular tension due to overuse or mechanical damage: When you knead a taut muscle, it begins to relax – and when a muscle has been damaged it may go into spasm (which again can be relieved a little by gentle manipulation and massage).

3. By inhibiting pain signals and closing the gate to pain: The Gate theory of pain was first put forward by two scientists called Wall and Melzack in 1965 (see above, p. 181). When a woman in labour has her lower back massaged and rubbed, the pressure of the strokes sends neurological signals which compete for transmission up the spinal cord to the brain with the neurological signals for pain. TENS (see p. 204) works on the same principle.

4. By psychologically relaxing the woman in labour: If a woman in childbirth is stressed, nervous or anxious, the amount of tension in her muscles increases, leading to a corresponding decrease in the level of natural opiate-like substances (endorphins) which are normally secreted to damp down labour pain. In the meantime, the anxiety can trigger production of adrenaline-like substances called catecholamines, which are usually only secreted in the second stage of labour.

Catecholamines stimulate the powerful expulsive contractions of the womb which push the baby out so it can be born. So if the mother's stress brings on an early release of catecholamines they will disrupt the first-stage contractions, which are designed to shrink the womb and pull up the cervix rather than to push (see pp. 30–33). This, and the fact that catecholamines are also thought to be pain-transmitters in their own right, is thought to increase the amount of pain a woman feels in childbirth.

This is why it is so easy for a cycle of lack of relaxation → anxiety → physical tension → increased pain perception to become established. And it can be difficult to break unless the mother relaxes again. Massage is one effective, gentle way to help her to do so.

5. By affecting the amounts of different injury chemicals the body releases: Why does it help a small child who has banged their knee to have the sore, reddened area rubbed better? One of the reasons, apart from the closeness and comfort touch can offer to someone of any age who is distressed, is thought to be that rubbing encourages the release of endorphins in the area.

The other reason is that rubbing brings about a fall in the level of histamines. When tissue damage occurs, histamine chemicals are immediately released; they have an inflammatory effect which makes the entire area sore. This inflammatory reaction, added to an increased blood flow to the area, makes it turn temporarily red.

So by reducing the level of histamines and increasing the level of endorphins in the area, rubbing produces two chemical changes which cause the pain to gradually die away.

HOW EFFECTIVE IS IT?

> Massage should certainly be considered a valuable resource in therapy as well as health promotion. Those who think otherwise have probably never had a good massage.
>
> *Dr David Sobel, Chief of Preventative Medicine at the Kaiser-Permanent Medical Centre, San Jose, California*

About 10 per cent of women use specific massage in their labours. Most midwives say they will usually rub women's lower backs at intervals as long as they are not too short-staffed. However, in the NBT survey women did not seem to see this as massage as such. Of those who used what they themselves regarded as massage, 90 per cent said they found it was either a 'good' or 'very good' method of pain relief.

Lower back massage and pressure seems to be especially helpful for women who are having back labours – feeling most of the pain of labour in their lower backs. This type of labour can cause great pain to the woman and can also be quite difficult to soothe.

A study of 500 women carried out in 1981 by the Obstetrics and Gynaecology Unit of Grand Rapids Osteopathic Hospital in Michigan looked at 500 mothers in labour who had particular back pain, and found that in 87 per cent of cases it was associated with their babies lying in awkward positions for birth.

The staff tried osteopathic techniques in lower back rubbing for half of them, and massaged less appropriate areas of the back for the mothers in the control group. Of the group receiving proper (osteopathic lumbar) massage designed to help labour back pain, 81 per cent reported relief. Further, the wrongly-massaged group needed about 30 per cent more doses of major narcotic pain drugs (Demerol) and 50 per cent more of the minor tranquillizing drugs often used for labour in America than the women having the 'real' back massage.

HOW CAN YOU HAVE MASSAGE FOR LABOUR?

You can, if you can reach comfortably, rub the part that hurts yourself. But this tends to tense up other parts of your body, and it never feels as good as when someone else is doing it for you.

It's possible to massage your own back by leaning back against a wall with a tennis ball wedged at the point where you are hurting, between your back and the wall surface, then rubbing yourself against it. Wooden-roller massage aids which you can buy from health shops or chemists can also be helpful.

Better still, get your partner or midwife to do some general massage for you:

- Ask them to rub, in a general way, right where it is hurting. They will need to use firm pressure which moves around a little. If the pressure is in exactly the same place all the time it will make the area very sore after a while.

- A gentle massage on the top of your shoulders and back of your neck is helpful. Tension will often collect in these areas when you are tensing against the contractions, eventually turning them painfully rigid.

- Long, firm strokes down each side of your spine with the masseur using alternate hands can also help. These strokes can extend down your hips and thighs, both areas where some women experience considerable referred pain.

- Having your buttocks kneaded firmly, as if someone were making dough with them, can provide a helpful counter-pressure to low labour backache. If your partner or midwife's hands are getting tired, they can use their fists, rolling the knuckles around the buttock backs and sides in slow circular movements.

If your partner would like to help you during your labour by massaging you, practise techniques and positions beforehand. It is difficult to do them for the first time when you are in pain, your partner is worried about you and you are both having to read notes or a book.

Stephen Sandler, Director of the Expectant Mothers Clinic at the British School of Osteopathy, and Consultant Osteopath to the Portland Hospital for Women & Children in London, teaches midwives and women's partners specific massage for labour. The techniques are based on gentle supported stretches as well as massage itself. His courses suggest four basic movements. You may find all of them helpful, or that a particular one or two are the most comforting:

1. The lower rib stretch: A woman in labour will be using the muscles where the ribs are attached to the thoracic part of her spine for pushing. Help keep these loose by sitting next to the mother, who also needs to be sitting, legs over the edge of her bed or chair, then:

   (i) Put one hand on her waist area and another on her shoulder of the same side
   (ii) Ask her to lean gently sideways into you
   (iii) As she does so, stretch the area between your hands.

2. The labour rub: A very simple and effective massage which can be done either as the woman sits, lies on her side, is on all fours (which many find very comfortable during labour), or leans across a chair back, pile of cushions, beanbag, edge of a bath or water pool. It provides counterpressure on her sacrum (the base of her back).

Cross your hands over the centre of her lower back (see fig. 10) and rub in rotating circles, rocking to and fro to use your bodyweight as you do so.

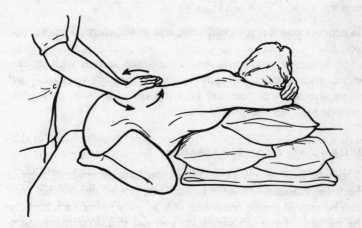

Lower back massage is a gentle, time-honoured way of helping women in labour to both relax and cope with pain.

3. The whole back stretch: The mother needs to sit on the edge of the bed or chair with her partner standing facing her. Then she crosses her arms in front, rests her head on the partner's forearms as they are held against his/her chest. The partner stands with one foot in front of the other, supporting the woman under her arms and rocks to and fro, stretching her gently upwards and letting go.

Don't be afraid to say what feels good and what does not. This is no time to worry about hurting someone's feelings, and most people would prefer to know if they are being helpful or not. Many men are only too willing to massage their partners in labour as they often feel very strongly they want to help, but need to have something specific to do. Instructions such as 'harder', 'more gently', or 'a bit to the left' are also important, and will help you get the maximum benefit from your massage.

WHEN CAN I USE MASSAGE?

Whenever you feel it would help, and at any stage of labour that you like.

If, however, you are having a caesarean section with an epidural, your partner will only be able to massage your head and front shoulders as you will be lying on your back, or slightly propped up, for the procedure.

WHEN CAN'T I USE MASSAGE?

It can be used at any time. But if you have an epidural in your back the masseur will need to take care not to disturb this. You can be moved gently onto your side so your lower back area can be rubbed. If you are sitting up you can still do gentle rocking and passive stretching and benefit from having your shoulders and neck rubbed.

There are no contraindications, so you can have any other method of pain relief with massage too.

Many women find some form of touch immensely comforting and helpful in their labours. However, it depends on how much they like being touched in general and also how they find they feel about being touched during childbirth. These are two different things, as sometimes women who like close physical contact such as hugging and cuddling will find that when they are in labour they prefer to be left to themselves, finding it irritating when someone does touch them. This may be so only for parts of the labour (often during the transition stage), or for the entire time.

HOW QUICKLY DOES IT WORK?

Depends on the type of massage. A general neck and shoulder massage for relaxation should start to relax you and reduce the pain within about 10 minutes. But if someone is rubbing firmly on a particular area that is hurting, this could begin to help within a minute or two because pleasurable touch sensations help to close the gate on pain signals.

HOW LONG DOES IT LAST?

The relaxation it brings can last for some time after the massage is over, and that in itself helps relieve pain.

Pros

- Can be very helpful for relieving pain.
- Comforting in other ways quite apart from the pain relief aspect. Sympathetic touch has the power to provide closeness, a feeling of physiological and psychological support, and encourages contact and communication between a woman and her birth attendants.
- Easily available.
- Can be used when you are becoming uncomfortable or when your back is aching in pregnancy.
- It can also be helpful in the first weeks or even months after your baby has been born, should you find you still have backache from constantly carrying/lifting an increasingly heavy baby, and from pushing a buggy every day (whose handles are usually designed at the wrong height). Post-delivery backache for as much as a year or so is common because your ligaments remain soft and stretchy for some weeks after the birth, which makes your back more vulnerable to injury.
- No adverse side effects for you or your baby.

Cons

- Unless you are massaging yourself (which can be difficult, and may not be especially satisfying and soothing even when you do manage) you need to have someone else to do it for you. They may not do it very effectively, or for as long as you would have liked.

- You can practise massage for labour for weeks with your partner and then, when it comes to the time, you may decide after all that you do not want to have anyone touching you more than is absolutely necessary.

HOW DO I GET IT?

Available everywhere – all midwives will do some massage for you as long as they are not understaffed and are able to spend some time with you. Your partner can always help you too.

If you want to find out more about massage in labour, see **Resources** for details of a book and a video on the subject. Classes like those run by the NCT and Active Birth movement will also cover it to some extent.

REFLEXOLOGY

WHAT IS IT?

Gently manipulating or pressing certain areas of the hands and feet to help correct illness, soothe pain and calm the mind.

HOW DOES IT WORK?

Reflexologists believe that there are areas called reflex points on the hands, face and feet (see fig. 11) which correspond to each organ and structure of the body – the inside of the ankle to the uterus, for instance. These reflex areas are thought to be joined to their corresponding body part via channels of energy through nerve endings just below the skin. They therefore form a map of the body, the right foot and hand reflecting the right side of the rest of the body, the left foot and hand the left side.

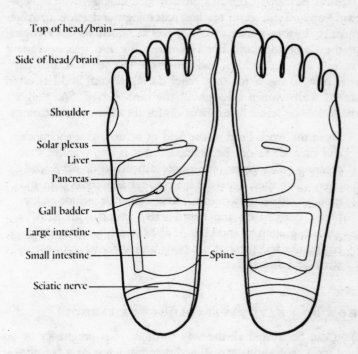

Reflexologists explain that this therapy works on the principle that different parts of the hands and feet correspond to different areas and organs of the body. By pressing and manipulating the areas which correspond, say, to the lower back or womb, reflexologists can help relieve childbirth pain and facilitate labour.

It is thought that by gently manipulating or pressing these areas, it is possible to rebalance the way the body works. Reflexology is not only used to treat physical problems, it is used by many therapists to help detect them too. If a particular reflex area of the hand or foot is very sensitive, this may suggest a problem developing in the organ or system which it corresponds to.

Fara Begum-Baig, formerly a biochemist who worked at the Medical Research Council's Neuroendocrinology Unit at Newcastle-upon-Tyne, now teaches reflexology and stress management to doctors, nurses and midwives at Addenbrookes Hospital in the Cambridge and Ely Hospitals. She also treats pregnant women with reflexology, and shows the mothers and their partners how to use it for pain relief during labour, and has often stayed with women throughout the birth herself. She suggests the following scientific explanation for the effects of reflexology:

> From the work I did in the field of neuro-active chemicals and their effect on the brain, I feel it is also possible that pressing reflex points stimulates subcutaneous nerve endings, which then cause the brain to release certain pain and mood-mediating chemicals. These chemicals include endorphins, encephalins and neuro-active amino acids such as glycine, glutamine and GABA, all of which act upon different tissues and parts of the body and affect its response to stress and discomfort.

HOW DO I HAVE REFLEXOLOGY FOR LABOUR?

You can be treated all the way through your pregnancy or go and see a professionally qualified therapist a few days before you give birth. A happy medium may be to see your therapist regularly for a few weeks before the birth. They can show you or your partner which areas to press – ask them to draw small Xs on your skin with an indelible pen or felt pen so it is easy to remember. Some will even be able to come with you to the birth, if that is what you would like (see **How do I get it?** below).

When actually treating you, they would press three or four times on the relevant points for about 30 seconds for initial effect, and repeat as necessary.

HOW EFFECTIVE IS IT?

There have been a number of published references in East European and Russian medical journals on reflexology in labour. The results of a study carried out by Drs Zharkin, Frolov and Kostenko evaluating a combination of reflexology and light anaesthesia for caesarean section appeared in the Russian journal *Akush Ginekol Mosk* in 1984, and in 1980 *Anesteziol Reanimatol* published the findings of Koraeva, Poluianova and Ustinova that reflexology proved helpful for reducing pain in the first stage of labour. And in 1981 an overview article by Zolnikov, Lapik, Ustinova and Shatkina, entitled 'Reflexology in the Obstetric Clinic' appeared in *Akush Ginekol Mosk*, which suggested that this therapy has a valuable place in obstetric analgesia.

In Britain, apart from an article entitled 'Reflex Zone Therapy for Mothers' published in *Nursing Times* in 1990 (which concluded that reflexology was helpful for women in labour) there has been hardly any published work on this as a form of pain relief in childbirth. This is because, where reflexology is concerned, it is difficult to set up the type of double blind placebo trials required for the validation of all new medical treatments by the orthodox clinical establishment. It has to be said, however, that some ordinary orthodox chemical treatments which have become an accepted part of obstetric and general medicine practice have not been validated in this way either. However, clinical research into the use of reflexology in general pain management is currently (1994) being undertaken at Cambridge University with NHS staff from Ely Hospital.

Some British midwives are trained in, and use reflexology. According to Fara Begum-Baig, from what she has seen, and from the comments of both midwives and mothers, it appears that reflexology can indeed be very helpful in labour for several things including pain relief. These include cervical dilation and speeding up labour itself.

Finally, according to Mo Usher, the President of the Association of Reflexologists, a recent British study of 37 mothers found that reflexology in late pregnancy reduced their need for pain relief in labours, and produced more rapid problem-free births.

The research was carried out in 1992–3 by a private practitioner with an especial interest in natural birthing and natural pain relief called Gowrie Mowtha, and a GP in Forest Gate, London. The mothers had 10 reflexology sessions beginning in the middle of their pregnancies and found:

- 2.7 per cent had an epidural (national average is about 20 per cent).
- Average first stage of labour times for mothers who had had the reflexology treatments were about five hours (compared with the usual 7 to 9 hours for first babies) and the average length of the second, pushing stage of labour – which for first-time mothers is anything between one and two hours – was reduced to 16 minutes.

Dr Mowtha is currently trying to set up a second, larger trial to confirm the findings of this initial smaller one.

Like most methods of pain relief, and especially most complementary methods, its effect is thought to be variable. However it has been reported that many women needed no additional analgesia after reflexology, and that midwives who have used this technique say first-time mothers had 'better than expected' labours as a result.

WHEN CAN I USE REFLEXOLOGY?

At any stage of labour, or post-delivery.

WHEN CAN'T I USE REFLEXOLOGY?

There are no recorded contraindications and no adverse effects on the mother or baby have been reported so far.

HOW QUICKLY DOES IT WORK?

It seems to begin to help within a minute or two, with the fullest effects felt up to 15 minutes later.

HOW LONG DOES IT LAST?

The beneficial aftermath may last for up to 24–48 hours afterwards.

Pros

- Can do it for yourself or your partner can be shown how.
- Relaxing and calming in its own right.
- Non-invasive, unlike acupuncture, which works on fairly similar principles but which requires the use of needles. Needs no other apparatus or ingredients you need to buy.
- Said to be useful for other labour problems, and also postnatally to help speed recovery.
- You can do reflexology for relaxation on newborn babies too, and apparently they like it.
- Does not involve taking anything internally.
- Appears to help the bonding process between mothers and their babies.

Cons

- Very important that a properly qualified therapist treats you.
- Initial cost – between £25 and £35 for a first session which would include a detailed medical history and interview, a treatment and instruction on which pressure points should be pressed for pain relief in labour.
- The fee for a therapist to be there for the birth, which might take several hours or be outside working hours, is likely to be £100 plus if you negotiate a flat fee.
- You would need to check with the Head of Midwifery Services, if you are having your baby in hospital, that there would be no problem about having your therapist there in a professional capacity (please see pp. 124–6).

HOW DO I GET IT?

To find a professionally qualified reflexologist, contact the Institute of Complementary Medicine or Association of Reflexologists (see **Resources**).

TRANSCUTANEOUS ELECTRICAL NERVE STIMULATION (TENS)

WHAT IS IT?

A method of pain relief which involves the use of four small electrode pads delivering a mild electrical stimulus to your back, which can help reduce the pain of contractions during labour.

Electricity has been used in medicine since AD 46 when a Roman doctor called Scribonius Largus used a fish called an electric ray (a member of the stingray family) to treat headache and gout. The shock from the ray stimulated the affected area and apparently helped to relieve some of the pain. In the 19th century it was also used, with very varying degrees of success, in the form of galvanism as a cure-all for a staggering variety of illnesses.

As used for women in labour today, the TENS system is small and light, with a control unit about the size of a cigarette packet. It is also easy to walk around with it if you wish, because it is battery operated.

TENS is also helpful for backache both before and after you give birth to your baby. Several other versions of the system are used in the NHS to relieve post-operative discomfort and to help deal with certain types of chronic pain such as arthritis, neuralgia, sciatica, and pain from damage to the back's discs.

HOW DOES IT WORK?

It is thought to work in two different ways:
1. Electrical stimulation at a rate of 2 Hertz (pulses) a second is thought to stimulate the release of endorphins, traces of which have been found in the fluid which bathes the spinal

cord. These are many times as strong as morphine, and so are potent painkillers. TENS is said to raise the body's endorphin levels if it is used continuously while labour pain is still mild.

2. During the contractions themselves, the TENS' electrical impulses travel down the fast-conducting A neural fibres to the brain, arriving there ahead of the pain signals from the womb which have to travel down the C nerve fibres which conduct impulses more slowly. This is called the Gate theory of pain. The TENS stimuli are literally closing the gate to pain so its impulses cannot reach the brain to register that something is hurting. (For a fuller explanation of the Gate theory of pain see p. 181.)

HOW DO YOU USE IT?

Place one pair of electrodes about halfway up your back on either side of your spine, and the other pair parallel to them on either side of the base of your spine, just above your buttocks (see fig. 12). This is far easier to do if they are the modern, self-adhesive type. Some older units have flat rubber pads, which need to have electro-conducting gel wiped on them before they are laid on your back and taped in place. It is possible to put them on yourself, but easier if a friend, partner or midwife can do it for you.

If you are not quite sure about where to place the electrodes, take them to your final antenatal appointment before your estimated delivery week and ask a midwife to mark four Xs on your back with an indelible pen showing where they need to go. Then if you have the self-adhesive sort, you can practise putting them on looking over your shoulder in a full-length mirror.

It is a good idea to practise a little with the TENS machine before you actually need it, so you can get used to using it and to the sensation it produces. Try wearing it for half a day, and practise pressing the buttons each time you have a Braxton-Hicks contraction. Many women also use it to help alleviate nagging backache late in their pregnancy, which for some can become severe and make it difficult to sleep at night.

Start using the TENs machine as early as possible in labour.

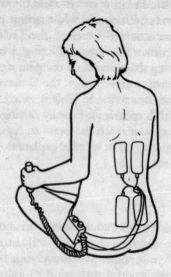

The TENS machine: four electrode pads are attached to your
back on either side of your spine. You control the delivery of
low-level electrical stimulation yourself with a push-button
hand-held unit. This competes with pain impulses and helps block
them.

This helps establish a good endorphin build-up. The other reason
is that if you wait until things become painful, repeated stimuli
travelling down well-worn neurological pathways will have
increased their reactivity to pain, and you will become progressively more sensitive to it; possibly so much so that when TENS
is eventually used you will not find it of much help.

Forestalling this potentially heightened sensitivity is called pain
prophylaxis (prevention). It is recommended by many top anaesthetists and pain experts, including a consultant anaesthetist at
University College Hospital who suggests, on the same principle,
taking a painkiller *before* you have a filling at the dentist's rather
than after.

You can adjust the machine to deliver high, medium or low

doses of stimulation, depending on how much pain relief you feel you need. When the machine is simply on you may be able to feel a constant gentle buzzing or mild tingling. If you boost the level of stimulation, this will increase, along with the machine's ability to reduce pain. As you turn it up, the buzzing becomes far stronger; unless you are having a contraction, it can feel a bit uncomfortable at high levels.

Leave the machine on all the time while you are in labour, and turn it up each time a contraction begins, turning it down again as each one finishes.

HOW EFFECTIVE IS IT?

About 5 per cent of women use TENS during childbirth, and it is available in roughly half of all maternity units. These women and their midwives seem to rate TENS higher than do doctors, many of whom regard it as 'essentially a labour-saving but fairly expensive way of rubbing someone's back'.

Estimates about how effective it is vary widely. The units' manufacturers and distributors claim a high success rate, and early trials in 1979 suggest it was helpful for about 80 per cent of women. In 1986, however, further trials contrasting dummy and real machines were far less positive, concluding that the machines did not even reduce the need for other forms of pain relief. Research at the pioneering Pain Clinic in Liverpool's Walton Hospital suggests that TENS only really helps about 10 per cent of their patients. However these people were sufferers from long-term chronic pain; labour pain is different because it is short-term and acute.

A study on the effect of TENS on women in childbirth at the Royal Sussex County Hospital in 1980 found that of 51 women tested 70 per cent found TENS useful

Of these, 8 out of 10 found it helped relieve their back pain, 7 out of 10 found it helped abdominal pain, 5 out of 10 found it useful during transition. But only 1 in 10 found it helped when they were pushing their baby's head out.

In the 1993 NBT survey however, 25 per cent of all the women who used it said it gave very good pain relief, another 25 per cent said it was of little or no help, and the rest were somewhere between – similar results to pethidine in fact.

Other studies have found TENS was no more effective than placebo.*

'I didn't think it was doing much. So I stopped pressing the button for the next couple of contractions, and immediately realized just how much it had been helping after all.'

'Good for the early to middle stages – but it did not seem to really touch the later stage at all. Also, the electrode pads and wires got in the way of my husband massaging my back.'

'It seemed ineffectual, apart from the psychological aspect of pressing the button.'

'Very good. I was able to cope until the late stages without gas and so felt I was more in control.'

WHEN CAN I USE TENS?

It is more effective in the early part of labour. Only about a quarter of the women who initially found it helpful say it continued to give effective relief in the second stage.

This is thought to be because much of the pain during the first stage is caused by the womb contracting and the cervix flattening and pulling up. These pain messages travel along the slow-conducting C fibres, so TENS electrical signals which are relayed

---

* Elisabeth Cluett, 'Analgesia in Labour: A Review of the TENS method', *Professional Care of Mother and Child*, Vol. 14 (1994), No. 2.

along rapid-conducting A fibres can partially block them before they reach the brain and register as pain.

But during the second, pushing, stage of labour, pain stimuli are coming more from the birth canal and the perineum stretching and the nerves in this area travel mostly along the A fibres and sending yet more signals down those same fibres does not help block the pain registration.

WHEN CAN'T I USE TENS?

- If you have a heart pacemaker
- If your baby's heartrate is being monitored electronically
- In water
- The electrodes must not be used on areas of skin which are broken or irritated.
- Check with an acupuncturist if you are also having electro-acupuncture.

HOW QUICKLY DOES IT WORK?

TENS begins to take effect almost immediately if used early in labour. But you will not feel the full effects for up to half an hour, as it takes endorphin levels this long to build up. Once established, these endorphins take some time to clear from your system, so the pain-relieving effects of TENS are often maintained for a while after the electrical stimulation has stopped.

HOW LONG DOES IT LAST?

The majority of women find it is of no help during their pushing stage. What pain-blocking effect it has earlier in labour will be lost straight away if the machine is turned off. But if it has been on long enough to generate a sufficient level of endorphins, there will be some reduction in pain for the hour or so it takes for these to clear from your system.

It is recommended that you keep using the machine and electrodes for an hour or two after your baby has been born to help maintain higher endorphin levels in your body. This may help relieve any discomfort you may feel afterwards, due for instance to being stitched (which some women say hurt more than the birth itself) or to general tissue stretching/soreness.

Pros

- Can be used right from the beginning of labour, and may mean you are able to stay at home if you wish for longer before leaving for hospital.

- Suitable for use in home births.

- Helpful for backache before and after labour too.

- Once correctly attached to your back it is under your own control, and you can increase its effect immediately if you need to.

- No reported adverse side effects for you or your baby.

- Does not affect your awareness.

- You can remain fully mobile and change positions or walk about as you please while using it.

- Compatible with all other forms of pain relief, apart from water, and possibly electro-acupuncture (check with acupuncturist).

- Can be useful when women have:

  (i)   internal examinations to see how far their labour has progressed; or membrane sweeps to encourage labour to begin (both these can be uncomfortable);
  (ii) Prostaglandin therapy to induce their labours, which can produce more frequent and, more painful contractions.

- Seems to be on a par with pethidine from an effectiveness point of view.

- If you do not like it you can just take it off immediately.

Cons

- Having paid to hire a unit, you may find it is of no help after all.

- Costs from £28 a month if you hire your own. If you do not, it is possible that the hospital may only have one TENS unit – and this might already be in use by another mother in labour when you need it.

- Does not usually work in the second stage of labour.

- Some women dislike the sensation it produces – though many who initially find it irritating say that this ceases to be noticeable when they are having painful contractions.

- To attach the older version, you need someone else's help, which can be difficult if you are in early labour on your own at home.

- You may find the wires a nuisance after a while, especially if you are having the sort of labour which means you need to go to the lavatory frequently.

- If used for a long period, it can cause some skin irritation around the site of the electrodes.

- It may have to be switched off if any electronic fetal monitoring is taking place.

HOW DO I GET IT?

About 50 per cent of maternity units have them, but many have only one or two, which means other women may be using them at the time when you need to. Ask what the situation is at your hospital. If you are having a home birth, ask if your midwife has one.

Alternatively you could hire a machine for a month. There are several companies which offer them for between £25 and £30 for four weeks (see **Resources** for addresses). If money is a problem, you could share one with another mother, perhaps someone you know from antenatal classes, who does not have exactly the same due week as you do (obviously the rental companies do not like you doing this as it means they make less money so – don't tell them).

POSSIBLE PHYSICAL PROBLEMS AFTER CHILDBIRTH

WHAT TO DO ABOUT DISCOMFORT OR PAIN AFTER CHILDBIRTH

You may experience no problems at all after the birth of your baby. But every woman's labour and post-partum period is different – there are no strict rules, just individual mothers and their babies. So you may equally well find that you have one, or perhaps more than one, type of discomfort or pain. If you do, this chapter is about the types of problem you may experience, and what you can do about them.

Whether the problem is minor or more severe, there is always something that you or the medical staff, or both, can do to make it very much better.

According to the Avon Longitudinal Study,* the most common types of postnatal discomfort/pain are:

Problem	Almost always %	Sometimes %
1st Painful stitches	9	40
2nd Backache	8	58
3rd Haemorrhoids	7	32
4th Headaches/ migraine	2	56
5th Shoulderache	2	28
6th Breast/nipple problems	1–2	34
7th Neckache	1	28

This may make it sound as if you are bound to have some form of pain after childbirth. You aren't. Almost half the women surveyed said they had *no* particular pain after giving birth.

* A large, on-going midwifery study in the UK.

However, the Avon Longitudinal Study's findings have been questioned by other researchers who feel these figures are too low. When the Aberdeen Maternity Hospital questioned about 200 newly delivered mothers in 1992, they found that 72 per cent needed some form of painkilling treatment the day after they gave birth. Of the first-time mothers, 77 per cent said their biggest problem was pain around their perineal areas from tears or stitches. Mothers who had had babies before reported that it was uterine cramps that caused them most difficulty. Even so, that still leaves nearly 25 per cent of mothers who reported no painful problems after the birth.

HOW TO GET HELP WITH PHYSICAL PROBLEMS AFTER CHILDBIRTH

Ask for as much help as you feel you need. If something is still not right, keep mentioning it to your midwife or GP. You are the best judge of whether your body is returning to normality properly or not.

Do not feel embarrassed about being a bit assertive, as no one is going to think any the worse of you because of it. All health professionals are there to help you and the other new mothers in their care. They recognize that this is a time when mothers *will* need help, and are almost always very happy to give it.

Now that hospitals have a policy of sending new mothers home sooner,* you may not be within reach of the midwives on the maternity ward 24 hours a day to help if any problems do develop. Therefore it can be useful to have as much information as possible about the potential causes and solutions for the most common types of postnatal pain, just in case you do find you need some help.

* In 1980 the average stay in hospital for a first-time mother following a normal birth was 7 days, in 1994 it was down to 2·4.

WHO TO GO TO FOR HELP?

While you are in hospital

Ask the midwives (especially about breast problems as they frequently have a great deal of experience in this area). If their advice does not help sufficiently, ask to see an obstetrician or another doctor who is a member of that obstetrician's team, and keep asking until you do. If you are not feeling up to making a fuss yourself, ask your partner to speak to the sister in charge of your maternity ward, in private.

If you are still unhappy despite the advice or reassurance that the doctor gives you, ask for a second opinion. You need not feel nervous or apologetic about asking for one, because it is your right to do so.

If you are seen during or soon after your labour by a doctor whom you like and trust, take down their name and ask whether, should any problems persist after you go home, you can come back and see them again. If they agree, ask how you can make sure of seeing them and not someone else – are there any special days when they are available in a postnatal clinic, for instance? Most doctors on maternity units work in the clinics at the hospital too, but it is best to check that your chosen doctor does. If this doctor is not going to be available, ask who they would recommend for you to come back and see instead with any problems. They will be able to suggest some appropriate colleagues, because good, sympathetic doctors tend to know who the others are in their hospital.

After you go home

Your community midwife will visit you daily for 7 or 10 days at least after the birth. Most will do so for up to a month if you are having difficulties. Your health visitor will be another good source of advice and support.

There may be a regular mother and baby clinic at your GP's practice; the staff there will have a special interest in post-partum problems and the right sort of experience to help you.

If you have a persistent problem, no matter how small it is, mention it forcibly to your GP when you go in for your 6-week postnatal check up. Ask to be referred quickly to a sympathetic consultant who has a particular interest in whatever is troubling you, to have it checked out – perhaps a consultant you met and had confidence in at the hospital where you had your baby (see above).

Hopefully it will be possible for your GP to refer you to the person of your choice on the NHS. If they are a fund holder, they may have a contract with this doctor's hospital. If not, there is sometimes money available in general practice budgets for what are called Extra-Contractual Referrals. They tend to be more willing to do this in the first part of their financial year than in the latter part when they are running out of money.

If you feel you are coming up against a brick wall with your GP, phone a help and advisory group or one of the campaigning organizations listed in **Resources**. They will be able to advise you and may even – off the record, because naming doctors for referral is considered advertising in the medical profession and is against their code of conduct – be able to suggest a good gynaecologist in your area who can help.

Private healthcare

This has advantages because:

- You can request that your GP refers you to a particular named doctor.
- 2. You will probably be seen more quickly. A private appointment, even for a new patient, can be arranged within a week to 10 days. On the NHS, you may need to wait several weeks unless the problem is acute.
- 3. The appointment would be at, or close to, a time convenient for you.

The big disadvantage is the cost. The fee will, on average, be between £50 and £100 for a first appointment. But, if you can afford it, going private may well be worth the money to at least get a diagnosis or clinical recommendation in writing, which you could then show to your NHS doctor if you could not afford to continue private treatment.

Common Problems

AFTERPAINS

SYMPTOMS

These range from an uncomfortable ache, like a mild period pain, to what some women describe as being as bad as labour pains themselves. They usually occur when you are breastfeeding, lasting for 5–10 minutes at the beginning of each feed.

Afterpains can be so mild as to be unnoticeable, or severe enough to make breastfeeding miserable, but fortunately they generally only last up to seven days even though it can take six weeks for your womb to contract back to its original size. They may not be noticeable after your first baby, but tend to become progressively sharper with subsequent babies.

CAUSES

Afterpains are caused by your womb contracting slowly back to its usual size (see fig. 13).

It is part of the restorative process which takes place in the womb muscles after each pregnancy. As the womb shrinks back to its normal size, any small tears that occurred in the muscle fibres during the powerful labour contractions are repaired by laying down small areas of fibrous scar tissue. These do not stretch or contract as easily as muscle tissue, and so may make the shrinking process uncomfortable.

Afterpains are not nearly so much of a problem for first-time mothers, as they are less likely to have these areas of scar tissue in the womb. They may also be especially uncomfortable if you have had your baby by caesarean (as 1 in 8 women in the UK do) because both your womb and abdominal wall will have had healing stitches in them. If this is the case, ask for stronger pain-killers, and try the self-help suggestions below (see also pp. 293–9 for ways to help you deal with the additional pain or discomfort that a caesarean operation may cause).

This discomfort is especially noticeable when you are

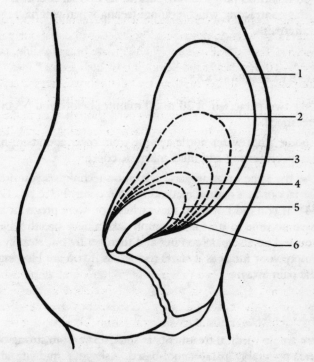

The uterus shrinks back to its normal size during the first six weeks after childbirth. When you experience afterpains (perhaps when breastfeeding), what you are feeling is this shrinking process.

breastfeeding because of surges in the hormone oxytocin. This affects two areas of your body, your breasts and your womb:

(a)   It acts on the breasts by causing the muscle tissue around the milk-producing lobes deep in your breast to contract, squeezing the milk up from these glands into the milk reservoirs just below your nipples. You might feel the process, which is called the let-down reflex, as a sharp tingling sensation, as needle-like pains or you may notice nothing at all.

(b)   In the womb, oxytocin causes its muscle tissues to contract, so it shrinks progressively back to its normal size. It is this contracting which you are feeling when you have afterpains.

SELF-HELP MEASURES

• Take two paracetamol 20 to 30 minutes before you begin to breastfeed.

• Cuddle a hot water bottle against your lower abdomen; heat has a comforting and mild analgesic effect.

• Use the same breathing and relaxation techniques you used for labour as a natural method of pain control (see pp. 129–34). If you did not learn these when you were pregnant and have no time to start now, simply take a deep breath when you feel an afterpain coming and then gently but steadily empty your lungs as it starts to bite, as if you are blowing the pain away.

TREATMENT

There are no medical treatments as such, apart from strong pain-killers, preferably paracetamol-based. Ask your midwife about these or, if you are at home, ring your GP and see if they can prescribe some for you which your partner can collect from the chemist on your behalf.

CONSTIPATION

SYMPTOMS

Hard, infrequent stools – infrequent meaning less than every three or four days; and hard meaning so firm that they feel pebblelike and are difficult to pass.

Women are often troubled by constipation during pregnancy, in the first few days after delivery, and frequently following a caesarean.

CAUSES

1. Pregnancy hormones: Constipation during pregnancy and after a vaginal birth is usually due to high levels of progesterone, a hormone which, amongst other things, relaxes muscle tissue so that the birth canal and cervix will be as flexible and stretchy as possible for the baby to pass through. But it does not act only on the pelvic area; it relaxes all muscles, including the smooth muscle fibres in the bowel whose usual function is to contract strongly, helping bowel waste pass down its length. This means that instead of being massaged and squeezed through the lower intestine, the faeces may get stuck, later becoming compacted and hard as the bowel absorbs its water content.

During pregnancy, progesterone levels build higher and higher, and though they begin to drop back to normal after the first few days after delivery, it takes a while for them to clear your system.

Post-caesarean constipation is also due to this. In addition, *any* abdominal surgery, including a C-section, can disturb the gut.

2. Perineal or vaginal repair stitches: If a woman has perineal or vaginal repair stitches, she may feel discomfort when she strains to pass faeces; and fear that they may also burst open. This can make her reluctant to try emptying her bowels, which will lead to a build-up of faeces in the lower intestine, and yet more constipation. Uncomfortable haemorrhoids developed during pregnancy and labour can make things even more difficult.

3. Recent eating and drinking patterns: Women tend not to eat during labour, and sometimes drink very little. They may not feel much like eating for a little while afterwards either. As a result they will have very little material in their gut to bulk out their stools and not much waste in their bowels to pass, so what there is may remain for longer than normal, becoming impacted and hard as its water content is absorbed by the bowel lining.

4. Pelvic organs returning to their normal places: Many women are not constipated after birth but will not move their bowels for about four or five days until all the organs in their pelvic cavity, including their lower gut, have recovered fully from being disturbed during labour.

SELF-HELP MEASURES

- A mild laxative (such as Lactulose, available from the chemist or pharmacist in hospital); this will not affect your baby if you are breastfeeding.

- A suppository to help loosen any faecal matter and also to lubricate the inside of the rectum.

- Keep taking sips of water during labour and drink as much water as you possibly can after delivery.

- Eat foods with some fibre in them as soon as you can. Fruit contains a good deal of water as well as fibre, and is easy to eat frequent small quantities of in hospital. Ask someone to bring you a small basket of apples, grapes (low fibre but high in water) and pears – or any other fruits that you specially like so you can keep dipping into it throughout the day. Banana sandwiches are also good.

- Do not strain for long on the toilet, but keep trying gently at regular intervals.

- If you are worried about stitches around your perineum, place a sanitary pad over them and hold it firmly but gently against the stitches for extra support as you push.

TREATMENT

If you are still unable to move your bowels after five days or so, either hospital staff or, at home, your GP, can first do a gentle enema of plain water for you. If this does not help, they should prescribe a stronger laxative or offer you a more powerful enema.

If you do have a stronger enema, it will suddenly, and without much apparent warning, become very difficult to hang on to the contents of your rectum, though the longer you can do so the better. If you are worried you might not reach the toilet in time, after about 15 or 20 minutes go and sit in there with a book, trying to retain the enema inside you for as long as you can. The longer you can hold it in for, the more effective it will be at relieving your constipation. This way at least you will be close to base when you need it.

You may find it helpful to continue to take a very mild laxative for a few days afterwards, until your bowels are functioning completely normally again.

DRY VAGINA

SYMPTOMS

Sometimes a problem for breastfeeding mothers, dry vaginae and labial tissues can cause discomfort when you make love and may also make it more likely that you develop itchy infections in the area. The former may not present much of a problem if you only plan to breastfeed your baby for a few weeks after it is born, and do not feel ready to make love then anyway. But some women breastfeed for many months and can find that a dryer than usual vagina can interfere substantially with their sexuality.

CAUSES

The hormones which help produce breast milk suppress oestrogen production, and it is oestrogen which helps to keep your vagina lubricated.

SELF-HELP MEASURES

You can buy KY gel or get a similar plain lubricant from the pharmacy. Vaseline can also help protect drier than usual labial tissue. The dryness will stop naturally when you are no longer breastfeeding.

TREATMENT

If the lubricant gel is not helping sufficiently, see your GP and ask if you can have some oestrogen cream to smooth on the entire area. Hormone cream is more effective from a lubrication point of view than plain gel.

A dry vagina and labia increases the likelihood of your developing infections ranging from bacterial vaginitis to thrush which will cause soreness and/or itching. Again, this can be avoided in the first place, or treated if you already have an infection, by creams and gels which can remoisturize the area, plus additional anti-fungal or anti-bacterial creams or pessaries to get rid of the infection itself.

Note: Sitting in a cool bath can help as a stop-gap measure until you can get to your GP, as some itchy genital infections can literally blow up overnight and become most uncomfortable very quickly. In the interim, use vaseline to stop dry and infected genital surfaces rubbing against each other.

LABIAL TEARS

SYMPTOMS

Your baby's delivery may have caused some small, shallow tears and grazes in the labia, the soft, fleshy lips around your vulva which enclose and protect the entrance to your vagina. These tears will be sensitive while they are healing, especially when you pass water, as urine can make them sting furiously.

PREVENTION

Water birth enthusiasts suggest that labour or birth in water may help reduce the likelihood of labial tears (see p. 184).

Homeopathic Arnica tablets or granules may reduce swelling and help healing, as can tincture of Hypericum.

TREATMENT

Large tears will be stitched (see pp. 272–7), but small tears generally heal by themselves within a few days as the blood supply to the area is very good.

SELF-HELP MEASURES

● Crushed-ice packs, wrapped in a clean cloth and held against the area. Do not hold the ice pack directly against the skin or you may develop ice burns. It is important to crush the ice so that it moulds itself comfortably to the contours of your perineum. If you have no crushed ice, packs of frozen peas or sweetcorn will do just as well, but smash out any frozen lumps in the pack first. The packs need constant renewal because they are less effective as they begin to warm up. Make sure no one tries to eat the contents (they will be in and out of the freezer, so may well be mistaken for a pack of frozen vegetables meant for cooking).

- Cooling sprays can help, though they may also cause stinging.

- Cold sitz baths. There is some evidence that these are more effective at reducing the pain for half an hour afterwards than warm ones – but very few people like taking cold baths.

- A warm bath. Soak for 20 minutes if possible, either in plain water, or in water with one of the following additives:

  i) Savlon, which can be soothing though it can make the bath quite slippery

  ii) Ten drops of Lavender essential oil from a good supplier (try brands like Neals Yard shops, Holland and Barrett or Tisserand Oils, see **Resources**)

 iii) A handful of coarse salt, enough so the water tastes quite salty

 iv) A herbal infusion made up of Loose Comfrey, Uva ursa and Shepherd's Purse (see **Resources** for shops where you can buy these). For one healing bath, put a big handful of this herbal mix in a bowl, pour four pints of boiling water over, stir and leave to steep for 30 minutes, stirring occasionally. Drain off the liquid and use this in your bath. Make one up if possible when you are still in very early labour at home, and put it in the fridge in a large lidded or stoppered container where it will keep for three days. Then, if you had your baby in hospital, ask your partner or a friend to bring it in as soon as possible afterwards, so you can use it there.

      Caroline Flint, President of the Royal College of Midwives, and herself an independent midwife, suggests adding an entire head of crushed garlic to the above mixture as it is both antiseptic and healing. The garlic may make the concoction smell strong, but it is anti-infective, and said to make the mixture even more effective.

- Pour water over your vulva when you pass water – keep a big glass or jug by the loo. You can also pour over some cold Comfrey tea (keeping the rest in the fridge for up to three days when not being used). Or use cool, diluted herbal bath mix (see above).

- Urinate in a bidet with the water spraying gently upwards, or in the bath (clean bath or bidet well afterwards though). Some women find it helpful to pass water standing in the bath, running cool water from a showerhead very gently over their perineal area as they do so, but it has to be done gently or the force of the water can hurt the perineum.

SWOLLEN VULVA

CAUSES

This is often the result of a long labour with strenuous pushing at the end but it tends to subside within a few days.

PREVENTION

Taking homeopathic tablets of Arnica before and during labour can help to prevent swelling, bleeding and bruising of all types.

SELF-HELP MEASURES

- Hold crushed ice packs against the area (this both helps reduce swelling and anaesthetizes slightly) but change them every 30 mins, as they warm up fairly rapidly. Do this lying down if you can.

- Bathe the vulva in a solution of 3 tsp salt to one tumbler of water.

- Lie down rather than sit when possible. Try to feed your baby while you both lie down together, as this will cut out several hours of sitting time. Ask your midwife to help you find a good position so your baby can latch on well, for although feeding lying down is very comfortable and restful for both of you, it can initially take a little practise.

- Wear large-size loose cotton pants to keep your sanitary towel in place rather than tight bikini pants.
- Choose a soft sanitary towel of cotton wool covered in wide-mesh gauze – and look for the packets marked 'Night Size' or 'Maternity Pad' – rather than the slimline variety.

PAINFUL BREASTS

Breastfeeding can be relaxing, easy, pleasurable, loving, exception-ally convenient and soothing for both parties. From the point of view of giving your baby both perfect nutrition and early protec-tion against infection, it has no equal. But it is not unusual to have a problem or two at the outset, nearly all of which can be resolved swiftly and easily if you get the right help. These may be related to feeding difficulties, postnatal breast pain, or a combi-nation of the two.

Unfortunately this help is not always available, because:

Women are being discharged earlier and earlier from hospi-tal after they have had their babies, frequently before they have had time to really try breastfeeding, let alone feel con-fident with it.

Community midwifery support, which is given to mothers for 10 days after a home birth, is stretched to its limits. Many midwives simply do not have the necessary time avail-able, and if a mother is having breast problems she may need more than one lot of advice or encouragement in a day.

Training for midwives and other health professionals in helping mothers to breastfeed and solve breast pain prob-lems is uneven. It is not unusual to get one set of advice (or even little advice) from your community midwife, a different verdict from your health visitor and yet another from your GP, which is both confusing and discouraging.

Getting help is therefore often a matter of knowing who to ask, and where to contact them. Not being able to get the right help when you need it, as soon as you need it, is a major reason why 65 per cent of mothers start off trying to breastfeed but only 25 per cent are still doing so four months after their baby is born.

> 'My breasts were lumpy and hard and hot. I hated the way they felt, I hated the way they looked – like alien growths on my chest, as if they weren't mine. It wasn't supposed to be like this if you breastfeed.'
>
> 'They were so sore I began to wonder why I was bothering when there were some perfectly good bottles downstairs.'

Breast pain, let alone the many potential 'how to' problems, can be enough to demoralize the most pro-breastfeeding of mothers. So even if sore breasts are not seen as clinically serious, finding ways to deal with the pain, and prevent it returning are very important.

There are several practical sources of advice and encouragement, including your community midwife, health visitor, and specialist help organizations like La Leche League, the NCT and the Association of Breastfeeding Mothers. They can all counsel you over the phone, and will also come and see you if they have a trained contact in your area – please see **Resources** for details.

A major part of the battle when it comes to overcoming initial problems and learning to breastfeed successfully is developing confidence in your own ability to do it. Caroline Flint believes that the peace, safety and familiar territory of the home gives a much more reassuring environment for a new mother than a busy hospital postnatal ward.

But it is vital that the mother gets all the help she needs at home, both from the midwife – who should visit daily and spend time checking technique and discussing problems – and from family, friends and partners.

Most people tend not to realize that breastfeeding is a demanding job in itself, not an extra to be slotted into an already tiring schedule. So it is vital to have time to take care of *yourself,* your own rest, comfort and diet in order to be able to feed happily and successfully. Get all the help you possibly can with your home and family. And let them know they cannot expect an especially well-run household for a while.

CAUSES

Discomfort or pain in the breasts can be caused by many different factors. However, they are all related directly to one or all of the following:

1 The action of breastfeeding itself.

2 The breast changes all newly delivered women experience in the first few days after they have had their baby, whether they are breastfeeding or not.

3 Infection.

Where there is any possibility that the problem is due to an infection, consult your GP immediately. They should see you the same day if you are trying to breastfeed and have a suspected breast infection.

The potential problems on the following pages are some of the most common causes of breast pain. Nearly all of them can be resolved either with self-help measures, medical treatment, or both, often within 24 hours of first developing symptoms. Your midwife or your health visitor will be able to advise you on any breast problems, so ask for help straight away.

BEATING BREAST PAIN

ABSCESS

SYMPTOMS

An abscess is an infected area filled with pus, like a large boil. Even if your breast no longer feels tender, you may notice that the skin over the abscess (which you cannot see) looks dimpled, like orange peel. Your milk may have a small amount of blood, or pus, in it. Neither will do actual harm to your baby, but they may make them vomit if they ingest a lot.

TREATMENT

There is no good self-help treatment for abscesses, so go and see your doctor as soon as possible. The area will need to be laid open and its contents removed. A hypodermic needle can be used for smaller abscesses, but you may need to have this done several times before all the pus has gone. Larger ones may need to be drained surgically under general anaesthetic. You would probably be given antibiotics as well.

You can continue to feed your baby while the surgical drainage incision heals, though some milk may seep out of the site, and it will heal more slowly. If you do carry on feeding, this will help prevent engorgement and further mastitis. Continuing to breastfeed with a healing abscess may not be easy, but it is perfectly possible, and good support from your nearest breastfeeding counsellor or doctor can make all the difference.

BLOCKED DUCTS

This is a small blockage in one of the delicate milk-carrying passages in each breast which brings milk from its storage and production place in the milk sacs up into the nipple. Sometimes it is possible to massage and express the blockage out gently by hand. Women report the blockages can look like a crystalline grain of sugar, a tiny lump or a very fine, short strand of spaghetti.

SYMPTOMS

- Pain in the blocked breast as your let-down reflex works, bringing milk from deep in your breast's milk sacs up to the surface of the nipple
- This pain may shift its position

- It tends to come on gradually
- You may have a slight temperature, but feel well otherwise
- A sore, lumpy area in part of your breast
- A reddish area on your breast – perhaps a stripe towards the nipple
- The breast may feel as if it has been bruised slightly.

RISK FACTORS

The following factors can all contribute to ducts becoming blocked:

a) Going to sleep in a position which squashes all or part of your breast – for example, sleeping on your front, or with an arm tucked underneath you and pressing hard against part of your breast.

b) A too tight swimming costume or bra. Underwired ones especially.

c) You may have skipped a feed for some reason, or be cutting down the number of feeds.

d) You may have had to hurry a recent feed so the baby did not take as much milk as usual.

e) You may have helped create more of a passageway for your baby to breathe while breastfeeding by pressing your finger against the breast. Although it sometimes looks as if babies' mouths and noses are pushed right up against your breast when feeding, so much so they surely cannot breathe properly, more than enough air invariably finds its way into their nose. If not, they would let you know by frequently stopping sucking to take a deep breath.

f) Your baby may have a minor illness such as a cold, which prevents them from feeding as well as usual. Tiny babies cannot suckle and breathe at the same time if their nose is blocked. This may mean they are taking less milk than usual.

PREVENTION

- Check your breasts daily for signs of blocked ducts. They are easier to unblock if they are very recent.

- Ensure you do not wear tight clothing or too tight bras.

- Talk to a breastfeeding counsellor, midwife or health visitor experienced in breastfeeding to see if there are other feeding positions you can try which may help avoid the problem.

SELF-HELP MEASURES

- Keep feeding your baby often from the affected side. Try doing so in the gravity position with your breast hanging downwards into the baby's mouth.

- If your baby is not keen to wake up, or is sleeping for longer periods at night, express milk to avoid your breasts becoming very full.

- Try a little massage using gentle, sweeping stroking movements right along the affected area towards the nipple. Soaping the breast and doing this with a wide-toothed or Afro comb can also be effective at helping to shift the duct's blockage – try this while having a bath.

- Do gentle arm-swinging movements to encourage good circulation in the area. Active housework with vigorous arm movements such as floor scrubbing, car and window washing have a similar effect.

- If there is a white spot, suggesting a blockage – perhaps of dried milk – on the nipple itself, this may be causing the blockage, so remove it gently.

DEEP BREAST PAIN

RISK FACTORS

If it is not caused by engorgement, blocked ducts, abscesses, or mastitis the pain may be due to:

(a) a muscle strain during delivery, especially a pulled back or chest wall muscle which is sometimes felt as breast pain during or between feeding in one or both breasts, depending on where the strained muscle is.

(b) An especially strong let-down reflex (release of milk from ducts deep inside the breast) felt as a sudden pain during feeding in one or both breasts. This can be a result of early engorgement, emotional stress and fatigue.

(c) Other factors likely to interfere with this let-down reflex include cracked and sore nipples, drinking a lot of coffee and smoking

(d) Thrush infection within the milk ducts. This can cause an intense, stabbing or burning pain either during or just after feeding and it may affect one or both breasts. You would need oral anti-thrush treatment, and so would your baby (see **Thrush**, below).

(e) Adhesions (old scar tissue) within the breast, perhaps from past surgery such as a lump removal or a blow on the breast.

SELF-HELP MEASURES

If the pain is due to back muscle strain, It helps to:

- Use pillows to support your baby's weight while you are feeding him.

- Support your own arms under the elbows with pillows when feeding.

- Again, when feeding, make yourself as comfortable as possible by leaning back in the chair and propping your feet up on a chair rung or low stool so your knees are higher than your hips, rather than leaning over your baby as you feed.

- Place a hot water bottle between your shoulder blades.
- Wear a well-fitting, very comfortable bra (see p. 242).

It will usually take less than a couple of weeks for the injury to heal. In the meantime, continue breastfeeding from the unaffected side.

If the pain is due to a very strong let-down reflex, consider trying:

- Any relaxation exercises which you may have learned during pregnancy for labour. If you have learnt relaxation, meditation or self-hypnosis, use this, with an affirmation at the end of it, to try and help calm the force of the reflex.
- Painkillers such as paracetamol, taken half an hour before you feed your baby.
- If your nipples are sore, this can make you tense just before, and when, your baby feeds from you. See pp. 249–55 for self-help measures to combat this.

Usually the let-down reflex becomes less noticeable after the first few weeks.

ENGORGEMENT

SYMPTOMS

If your breasts feel volcanic – hot, painful, skin taut and stretched to bursting point – the problem is usually engorgement.

Most mothers find their breasts swell up uncomfortably when their milk is coming through for the first time – changing from colostrum, the nourishing clear fluid which is the forerunner of full white milk. But some mothers find that their breasts are too tender to touch at all, or feel as if they are about to explode on the third or fourth day after giving birth. Others are able to feed their baby with no problems for the first few weeks, and then suddenly, their breasts become tender, hot, hard and swollen. Both problems are labelled engorgement of the breasts, but there are two types.

> 'My breasts felt like twin pressure cookers.'
>
> 'Even though they were sore, it seemed miraculous to have breasts like these – I have been size 32A all my life I could not stop looking at them.'

The swelling up of your breasts during *primary* engorgement is due to a surge of the milk-making hormone prolactin, which causes your breasts to be flooded with blood and fluid to begin milk production. The swelling may be just around the nipple area or the entire breast. Primary engorgement takes place in the first few days after your baby's birth and settles down rapidly.

Secondary engorgement develops later, perhaps after you have been feeding your baby perfectly well for some while. It is caused by a build-up of milk within your breasts and it can happen if the milk is not being removed at the same rate as it is being made. This produces distension within the milk sacs inside the breast and a rising internal pressure. If this pressure becomes great enough, it can also force some of the milk out into the surrounding tissue, producing inflammation of the breast.

Is it engorgement or fullness?

Breast fullness is *not* the same thing as clinical engorgement though the terms are often used as if they meant the same thing. Fullness happens for almost every woman who has just had her baby. However, while it may be uncomfortable, it does not make it difficult for the baby to feed, nor does it cause the mother pain. True engorgement hurts and can give you a temperature.

Engorgement vs Fullness: what is the difference?

Fullness	Engorgement
Seldom hurts as such, though it can be uncomfortable	Breasts will actually hurt

It is possible to press and compress the breast gently	Breasts feel rock hard, and you will not be able to compress them
Breasts are not so swollen that they prevent the baby feeding	Breasts so swollen that it is hard for baby to feed, which in turn can lead to more engorgement
Temperature normal	Your entire body temperature a degree or two higher than usual

RISK FACTORS

Primary engorgement

The most common reason for breast fullness is that the baby is not quite latched on properly to your breast. This is not always immediately obvious and it may only need a very small adjustment of position to put it right. According to breastfeeding expert, Cambridgeshire midwife Chloe Fisher: 'A tiny adjustment can make a world of difference.'

The other very common reason for engorgement of both types is delay in putting the baby to the breast for the first time. This is why breastfeeding experts recommend letting him or her suckle as soon as possible after birth – within the first hour if you can.

One of the reasons that women who had their babies by caesarean section may find they are more likely to have engorgement problems than mothers who delivered their babies vaginally is that it can take time to find the most comfortable way to breastfeed (or bottlefeed) your baby if you have abdominal stitches. And if you had a general anaesthetic, both you and the baby may feel groggy and sleepy for several hours afterwards. In fact, your baby may respond to receiving some of the anaesthetic drugs via your placenta by being rather sleepy and showing a disinclination to suckle for several days afterwards.

However, now that some caesareans are done by spinal or epidural anaesthetic, babies tend to be put to their mother's breast much sooner than if they had been delivered under general anaesthetic. This also means that neither they nor their mothers are hampered by the aftereffects of a GA, which can make early breastfeeding more difficult.

Secondary engorgement

Often this comes about because the baby's intake is reduced or the normal feeding pattern is disrupted, so milk builds up in your breasts. Common causes can include:

- Giving extra fluids to the baby besides your own breast milk, such as water and dilute juices or formula baby milk, because this can reduce the amount of milk they need from your breasts.

- Using dummies.

- Not feeding often enough.

- Feeding for very short periods only. But what is a short period to some babies may be a long time to others and it is almost impossible to make a tiny baby prolong its feed if it feels it has already drunk enough.

- Feeding from one breast only at each feed may be a factor. But equally, many women find they get on very well by alternately feeding their baby from one breast at one feed, and the other at the next. See what works best for you and your baby.

- When the baby first begins to sleep through the night, you may get an erratic pattern for weeks or even months of having to feed them every three hours one night, then not for the first five or six hours the next, and not for eight the next, then back to every three hours again. This can mean that sometimes your breasts will be producing more milk than is taken from them, and they may become engorged because of this.

- If you feed a great deal for a short period then drop back to more widely spaced feeds. This may be to give comfort because your baby is unwell for a few days, or almost continuously for comfort and calming over a long car or plane trip.

If either type of engorgement is not dealt with, it may develop into Mastitis (see below).

PREVENTION

Feed early.
Start as soon as you can after your baby has been born.
Feed often. As often as possible.

> 'Just a bit of extra feeding did the trick. It was so simple, but it took my health visitor to suggest it. I was relieved but I still felt like it should have been me that thought of it.'

TREATMENT

Medical treatment would be purely supportive, unless your breast pain was due to milk coming through for the first time and you had already made a decision that you did not want to breastfeed your baby.

If this was the case, you might be offered milk-suppressing hormonal drugs like bromocriptine which are effective but may make some women feel sick. To help avoid this nausea, take the first one before you go to bed at night (hopefully your baby will be asleep for two or three hours too) so you sleep through the worst of the effect of this dose. There is also a possibility of rebound engorgement after you have finished the medication, by which time you will be at home.

SELF-HELP MEASURES

If you do not wish to breastfeed

The old-fashioned treatment of binding your breasts up firmly with a wide, soft, crepe bandage for a few days to support them well until the engorgement has ebbed away of its own accord is still popular, as is its modern equivalent, a well-fitting, very supportive maternity bra. If either are too tight, or if the bra does not fit well or has supporting underwiring, it may encourage mastitis.

If you would prefer a bra rather than a bandage, it is very important to buy it from a store which has experienced and well-trained bra fitters (see **Resources**) who can estimate the size you would need to use very carefully. It is astonishing the temporary size change breasts can undergo during initial primary engorgement, and it can be difficult to judge this accurately without some expert advice. A bra bought at a guesstimate from a chainstore with limited cup-size range could turn out to be of little help.

'I didn't want to breastfeed Luke, though everyone said I ought to. I'd tried before with Mark, who's now four, and I just did not like that suckling feeling, it felt too animal like. The bandaging up of my breasts was very comfortable, but they did seem to be reproaching me for my decision not to use them'.

If you do want to breastfeed

Buy a comfortable, supportive maternity feeding bra. The NCT and La Leche offer their own mail-order range of good ones (see **Resources**). However it is best to visit a shop a few weeks before the baby is born to be sized accurately by a trained fitter; then you can if you wish order the styles you like via catalogues.

Before each feed:

- A warm bath to relax the distended skin of the breasts. Some women take the baby in too and feed them while reclining in warm water.
- Cool compresses – cold flannels would do fine – on your breasts between feeds, then warm compresses or flannels at the start of a feed.
- Very gentle self-massage on your breasts working from the

chest wall towards the nipple in a soft circular motion with your fingertips. Again, a good place to do this effectively is in a warm bath or shower.

- Chill some large Savoy cabbage leaves (the dark green, crinkly variety) in the fridge, then crush slightly with a rolling pin – which is said to release the enzymes they contain. Placed over your breasts inside your bra, these are surprisingly soothing. Many midwives and mothers recommend them. However, the only clinical trial to see if this really does help (done in South Africa, 1993) found the cabbage leaves didn't appear to help with the actual pain – but that they seemed to mean women breastfed their babies for longer after delivery.*

- Painkillers like paracetamol taken 20 minutes before feeding. Do not take codeine, as this can cause constipation and many women are constipated anyway after giving birth; or aspirin.

> 'They were burning hot, and so large they felt fit to burst. The only thing that helped were flannels and cabbage leaves. I don't know what I must have looked like, sitting in bed in hospital with everyone else's visitors coming and going, and these green frilly bits poking out of my nightie, but I was beyond caring.'

During feeding: if you are still rather engorged, try:

- Feeding your baby more often, and for longer periods.
- It may also be worth asking your local midwife or breastfeeding counsellor to come and see you breastfeed, to make doubly sure your baby is latching on properly to your breast, and therefore taking plenty of milk from it. If they are not, this means that too much milk is being left behind, causing over-fullness in your breasts.
- Speak to your midwife or breastfeeding counsellor about how

* Nikodem, Daniger, Gebka *et al*, *Birth*, Vol. 20, pp. 61–4.

often you are feeding the baby, and discuss whether a change in the pattern might help.

- If the engorgement happens during the first days you are breastfeeding when the flood of blood into your breasts is making them hard and tender, try letting your baby suckle at them fairly often to help relieve the pressure.

- If your breasts are too swollen for the baby to feed from easily, or so full that milk gushes into their mouth making them splutter and choke, try expressing a little first so the breast is softer and easier for him to feed from. The baby will take more milk if it is comfortable when feeding, and this will help reduce the pressure which has built up inside your breasts.

- If you use a breast pump, make sure it has a very comfortable action. The electric breast pumps in hospital are helpful here (you can also hire them via the NHS or NCT if you are at home). Alternatively, contact either the NCT or La Leche for suggested types you can buy. Not all pumps are the same as some have a suction action like a Hoover which can be painful on already sore breasts, others are ineffective. If you have a battery- or hand-operated one and you are having trouble getting your milk flowing with it, try sitting in a warm bath and using it. Alternatively, very gentle hand-expressing, again in a warm bath, can be a more comfortable option.

- Nipple shields, which are flexible artificial nipples placed over your own when the baby feeds from them, are sometimes suggested on the grounds that it is easier for a baby to latch on to these than to a very swollen nipple. But this has its drawbacks, as some breastfeeding counsellors say it may contribute towards nipple confusion if the baby is still in its first three or four weeks.

  Nipple-confused babies are said to feed less effectively and may refuse your breast altogether, which will make your engorgement even worse. Also the amount of stimulation your nipples are getting through a shield is reduced by over 50 per cent with the thicker older types, and by about 20 per cent with the new, very thin latex varieties – which again would eventually reduce your milk supply.

MASTITIS

Mastitis is an inflammation in the breast. There are two types, infective and non-infective.

Non-infective mastitis: This may follow on from a blocked duct which has not been promptly treated.

Infective mastitis: This is not very common in the UK. But if it does develop, it is often caused by an infection (frequently bacteria from the baby's nose or from the mother's own skin) which has found its way in via cracks in sore nipples.

SYMPTOMS

- A temperature.
- Small red patch on your breast, usually on one side only and in the upper, outer part.
- A sore area on your breast, but nothing visible.
- Feeling tired.
- Feeling as if you are coming down with flu (fatigue, headache, aching muscles).
- You may also just feel generally unwell.
- Usually the flu-like symptoms arrive first, then a hot, red area on your breast.

Is it a blocked duct, or is it mastitis?

If you have a plugged breast duct, one of the delicate milk ducts has become blocked with solidified milk. This is often confused with mastitis. However there are clear differences between the two:

Blocked duct	Infective mastitis
Mild pain	Intense pain
Pain comes on gradually and may shift its position	Pain comes on suddenly and stays in one place
You may have a slight temperature	High temperature
You feel generally well in yourself	Your breast is hot, red and swollen

RISK FACTORS

In 1990 the *Journal of Human Lactation* published the findings of a study of 161 new mothers. According to this study, the commonest reasons mothers themselves mentioned for their mastitis were:

1 Tiredness (24 per cent)
2 Stress (22 per cent)
3 Plugged milk ducts (17 per cent)
4 Change in the number of feeds (15 per cent)
5 Engorgement (10 per cent)

Other factors which are thought to increase your chances of developing mastitis include:

- Cracked nipples
- Tight bras
- Sleeping so that one of your breasts is heavily compressed in one area or all over
- An infection such as colds or flu in the family
- Producing too much milk. If your baby does not want all the milk your breasts are making and they still feel uncomfortably full even after a feed, express some milk to relieve the pressure.

It is thought that up to one in three women who breastfeed their babies for a long time will develop mastitis at some point. It usually happens during the first few weeks, but a third of cases occur after the baby is six months old, and a quarter after the baby is a year old.

TREATMENT

As a first-line treatment, try some of the self-help measures listed below. If these are of no help, ask to see a doctor, who will probably prescribe a broad-spectrum antibiotic. Check that it is one which would not affect your baby and is compatible with breastfeeding.

Mastitis which returns at intervals

It helps to:

- Always take the entire course of antibiotics prescribed otherwise you run the risk of recurrence. You would need at least 10 days' worth. If the problem does return despite a long course of which you took every pill, it is likely you have been given the wrong antibiotic.

- Suggest the doctor takes a sample of your milk and a throat culture from your baby to see exactly which bacteria is causing the problem so your GP can give you a more appropriate treatment.

SELF-HELP MEASURES

If there is some doubt as to whether the mastitis is really being caused by an infection, before taking antibiotics, try:

- Breast massage, encouraging any lumpy areas of your breast to drain by stroking them towards your nipple. Many women find it is easiest to do this in a warm shower or bath.

- Continuing to breastfeed as often as you can. Express milk if the baby doesn't want it all. Mastitis clears up faster if your breast is not allowed to become over-full.

- Try expressing some milk anyway, because if the problem is being caused by a plugged duct, it may be possible to encourage this to clear. Some mothers report a thick, yellowish looking plug or lump of material emerging after gentle milk expression, which clears the duct.

- Ask a breastfeeding counsellor (see **Resources**) your local midwife, health visitor or a friend who is or has breastfed her babies to come and see you to help you check that your baby is latched on to your breast in a good position. If they are not, this can reduce the amount of milk your baby is able to get from your breast, and again, lead to mastitis. If your breasts still feel full after feeding, this may be the problem.

- Check for, and treat, cracked nipples.

- Resting in bed if and when you can, even if it's only for half an hour at a time. Get as much help as you can with everything from cooking to shopping and child care from as many sources as necessary until you are better. Ignore things like housework as far as you possibly can. This may go against your usual instincts but in fact, it can wait, because your health is far more important at the moment.

Breastfeeding at night: how to make it easier

You may have little choice about feeding often at night as well as daytime, as newborn babies tend to want to breastfeed every two or three hours. This can be exhausting as it would mean you only have sleep in one to two hour snatches at first.

It can help to take the baby into bed with you so you only need to roll over rather than get up each time. Or have a baby basket right next to and on a level with your bed, so you can just lean over and bring them into bed for each feed, keeping them snuggled against you, or tucking them back into their basket again afterwards without leaving your own bed. Modern, more absorbent nappies and good protective barrier nappy creams also mean you do not have to get up and change them after each feed at night either, unless they are not just damp but wet or soiled.

If you are feeling run down and are vulnerable to infections in general, have a medical check-up and ask them to test you for anaemia. It might also be a good idea to consult a nutritionist or homeopath about how to improve your immunity to infection and general vitality (please see **Resources**). There are several good over-the-counter tonics, iron and multi-vitamin preparations which may help, such as Floradix, available from health shops. If you are taking iron tablets drink a glass of orange juice or take some vitamin C at the same time, otherwise you will not absorb the iron.

SORE AND CRACKED NIPPLES

SYMPTOMS

Your nipples may feel very tender to touch, making it difficult for you to feed your baby. Other symptoms of sore nipples, apart from pain, include:

- Red, sore looking nipple for light-skinned women
- Very shiny looking nipple for dark-skinned women
- A blister on its end
- A white area on its end
- Small cracks in and round nipples
- Small amount of blood in the cracks

It is also possible for your nipples to feel very sore, yet show no physical sign of any damage.

Levels of discomfort vary from barely noticeable to extremely painful, though it should disappear completely when your nipples become used to being suckled upon, within two or three weeks.

Between 80 to 95 per cent of breastfeeding women experience temporary nipple soreness of some sort, with a quarter of these saying their pain was extreme.

RISK FACTORS

Despite old wives' tales to the contrary, clinical studies have now shown it has nothing to do with the colour of your skin or hair (redheads and the fair-skinned have always been said to be the most vulnerable). Nor with whether you prepared your nipples for the mild mechanical trauma of breastfeeding while you were still pregnant by regularly rubbing them with something slightly abrasive like a flannel or towel.

Some degree of nipple soreness is highly likely during the first seven days, and is caused by a combination of the unrelieved pressure building up inside your breasts and the baby suckling at your nipples, sometimes for long periods, several times a day.

Many babies will want to suckle a good deal for comfort and closeness in the first few days, even if they are only getting small amounts of colostrum rather than several ounces of milk each time. Nipples are not used to this much stimulation nor to being kept damp for long periods, so they may initially react by becoming sore until they toughen up a little. Towards the third and fourth day, a newborn baby may start suckling for increasingly long periods as they become hungrier. Fortunately this is also the time that your small amounts of rich colostrum will give way to larger amounts of milk.

'It was like someone had rubbed chilli peppers on my nipples. It hurt even to touch them gently, let alone feed Kimberly with them. I knew I should keep at it for her sake, until the infection went, but I dreaded her feeding times and would sit there flinching, with tears running down my face.'

'Once I had some antibiotics there was a big improvement in 24 hours – and the pain disappeared almost as quickly as it had come.'

Why damp nipples become sore nipples

When the skin is wet (as the nipple is when a baby is feeding from the breast) it absorbs moisture and swells up. Rapid air drying causes it to shrink again irregularly. The resulting tension on the skin can cause it to crack. This is why some sore nipple treatments which concentrate on speeding up the drying process – such as using hair dryers on a cool setting to dry the nipples – or even ordinary air drying in low humidity areas, might make them crack even more.

Using emollient creams will encourage them to dry slowly and gently, and help avoid any small scabs forming.

Mothers who do develop sore nipples say the problem usually reaches its peak between the third and sixth day after delivery and then improves rapidly. If it persists after the first week, there may be a number of reasons why, involving both the mother and her baby, because breastfeeding is a two-person activity.

PREVENTION

1 Latching on: The most important way to help avoid sore nipples is to make sure your baby is properly latched onto your breast.

Your baby's cheeks should be rounded outwards, a good area of nipple and areola in their mouth, their lower lip curled outwards and downwards – and there should be no audible slurping noises. If there are they suggest he is sucking his own tongue, or not creating a tight seal around your areola.

Do not take too much notice of advice about having to get all the areola round your nipple in the baby's mouth. It is only relevant if your areolas are fairly small – about the size of a 2p piece. This is physically impossible if they are large, and many women's are. Try and get the bottom part of your areola in, with your baby's bottom lip curled down and back (see fig. 14).

Ask your midwife, health visitor or local breastfeeding counsellor to come and see you breastfeed, so you can make sure the positioning is exactly right, and alter it slightly if need be.

2 Resting and expressing: Instead of breastfeeding directly, express milk to put in a bottle for your baby's feeds for a couple of days. It is often easier to express milk sitting in a warm shower or bath.

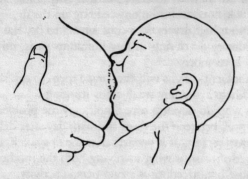

One of the most effective things you can do to help avoid painful nipples when breastfeeding is to check your baby is latched on to your breast in the right way. When a baby feeds, they need to take your whole nipple deep into their mouth, gums fixing to the base. They also need to take in a good section of the areola (but not, as is often advised, the whole lot – with large areolas that's physically impossible).

You can keep breast milk chilled in a fridge for up to two days before use. But you must put expressed milk into a sterile lidded container in the fridge straight away. If you are using a pump or drip catcher, any parts in contact with the breast or milk must also be sterilized daily.

3 Easing your baby off the nipple: When they have finished sucking and you want to take them off your breast but your nipple is still firmly in their mouth, first gently slide your (clean) little finger into the corner of their mouth to break the suction. If you pull your baby off the nipple, that can make them sore very quickly. Usually, babies will let go themselves when they have had enough and will not need to be taken off – unless they have fallen fast asleep still holding tight.

4 Protect your nipples from being constantly damp: If the nipples are allowed to remain damp, this can have a similar effect to leaving a wet nappy on a baby's bottom for too long – soreness and redness. Instead, dry your nipples gently with soft tissue every time you have finished feeding your baby.

Protect your nipples from being kept wet by leaking milk. Often the one you are not using will leak as you feed from the other side. It may help to:

(a)   Use a drip-catcher device. They look like small plastic flying saucers with a hole in the middle for the nipple and a pouring lip on one side. You can get them from large branches of Boots, or specialist medical suppliers such as John Bell & Croydon (see **Resources**). Often two or more ounces of breast milk can be collected this way, and it may be useful for mothers who want to express milk for their baby's use later – perhaps for a partner who is doing a night shift. After each feed, you can save one or two ounces of breast milk in a sterile bottle kept in the fridge.

(b)   Place a dry breast pad over the nipple you are not feeding from, keeping it in place with your bra. Change it, and dab that nipple dry afterwards with a dry tissue if the baby does not suckle from it on this particular feed.

(c)   Keep damp breast pads or soggy bras from touching the nipple itself by using the circular heads of two small plastic tea strainers inverted over your nipples, held in place by your bra. A large breastpad could go on top of that. Your nipples may then leak milk but it would not remain in contact with them because of a damp breast pad – the latter would merely stop any leaks from wetting your bra.

5 Avoid using soap or any form of detergent to wash your nipples: Plain warm water is fine.

Other useful ways of healing/preventing sore nipples:

• Use a cotton bra rather than a nylon one.

• Avoid breast pads with plastic backs. They prevent milk leaking through onto your bra and clothes effectively, but do so by keeping the moisture in against your breast.

- Try not to let your baby drag downward on your breast and nipple. Support them well from below instead. Bring your baby *up* to the nipple rather than letting him pull it downwards towards him.

- Feed from the least sore side first.

- If your nipples are very cracked, a thin latex nipple shield (available from the chemist) may help protect it while it heals, though you will find feeding takes a bit longer, and if you use shields for too long they may also eventually reduce your milk supply.

- When possible, expose sore nipples to fresh air by sitting with the cup flaps open (but with the supporting bra still in place).

- Try rubbing some of the richer hind milk, which comes at the latter part of each feed, into your nipples and areolas as it can be healing and moisturizing in its own right.

- Use a soothing cream which also forms a protective barrier over nipples to keep them from getting damp between feeds. Try something like Kamilosan, which contains the soothing plant extract Calendula (available from most chemists). In the first few weeks, whether your nipples are sore or not, it might be useful to put barrier cream on after a feed as it can prevent them becoming so. Plain lanolin cream may also be helpful here, but check it is definitely pesticide-free first. Hypoallergenic lanolin cream for clinical use may be the best option (available from your GP, and also from the La Leche League).

- Tea bags. This is an old, traditional remedy, but many practitioners and midwives say putting cold, previously used tea bags on sore nipples does indeed help because they contain tannic acid. There is no clinical evidence that it works, but because the substance is a mild astringent it may help reduce inflammation. It is sometimes advised as a home remedy for sunburn for the same reason.

- Keep feeding your baby as often as necessary. Hospital staff frequently tell mothers with sore nipples to limit feed times to give their nipples a rest, but in reality this may put off the time when they become sore until after they have gone home from hospital.

- Avoid using breast pumps too much. With many types, their action is so strong it can contribute to nipple soreness.

THRUSH

If your nipples are persistently sore, go to see your GP to check you do not have a thrush infection. Babies may sometimes be born with this in their mouths or they may develop it after birth, and they can pass it on to you when they feed.

SYMPTOMS

Check your baby for:

- White, irregular-shaped spots in the mouth that look like milk curds but cannot be wiped away with your finger
- Soreness around their anus or vulva, which may be thrush infection.

Check yourself for:

- Itching nipples
- Reddened sore nipples and areola
- An inflamed redness which may spread beyond your nipple and areola
- Vaginal thrush. Symptoms include: redness/itching around your vulva, and a curdy white but non-offensive smelling discharge from your vagina
- Oral thrush (white spots in your mouth)
- Anal thrush infection (again, redness and itching in the area).

'They kept giving me antibiotics because my nipples were so sore and red. The trouble was that it was thrush. Once I got some antifungal cream, and had some medication for Natalie, it cleared up really fast. I am still feeding her eight months later.'

RISK FACTORS

You should avoid tight nylon pants, tight jeans or lycra leggings, as these can make it more likely you'll suffer from vaginal thrush.

Mothers with a dry vagina or labia (eg if breastfeeding) are also at risk.

TREATMENT

You would be treated with topical cream, or cream and an oral treatment; your baby would be given an oral antifungal medicine.

If you are having sex with your partner, they will need to be treated too and you would need to use condoms to have intercourse until you were both clear. Thrush tends to be symptomless in men, so they can continually keep passing it back to you without realizing it.

See also caesarean sections and thrush, p. 296.

BACK PAIN

A common place to feel back pain after childbirth is at the point where your spine joins your pelvis: the sacroiliac joint. You normally feel it over the joint itself, which lies directly under the two dimples on either side of your lower back, just above your buttocks.

SYMPTOMS

It may start as a gnawing ache or sharp occasional twinge just after your baby is born which you hope is going to go away on its own – as it well might. Alternatively, it might persist so that you are in intermittent or constant pain which can range from uncomfortable (so you try to avoid making certain movements which bring it on) to the downright immobilizing.

RISK FACTORS

Most women develop backache to some extent in the days or weeks after they have had their baby, perhaps as a continuation of postural problems which developed while they were pregnant, or because of the position they laboured and actually gave birth in.

Problems which develop during pregnancy

- Change of posture to accommodate the growing baby, which often involves hollowing out your lower back, pushing your knees back and rounding your shoulders.

- Softening of the ligaments holding all your joints together, including those in your back. The rising levels of pregnancy hormones does this, but it is necessary as it helps your entire pelvic area to become supple and stretchy enough for the baby to pass through when it is being born.

- Abdominal muscles weakened by having stretched so much during pregnancy – a waist measurement which starts off at 26in usually reaches 46in. Your abdominal muscles help to support your back, so a weak abdominal wall means a more vulnerable back.

During labour and delivery

- Adopting any position which puts put excessive strain on your back: for example, sitting for hours, then giving birth with your knees up and back inadequately supported (as may be the case with an epidural; see pp. 86–7). Early research suggests that mobile epidurals lead to fewer back problems (see p. 90).

- Very long, tiring labours. Tired muscles are more susceptible to being strained and torn, as any sports medicine specialist or athlete knows to their cost.

- Straining the back during the pushing stage.

- General anaesthetic. Aberdeen Maternity Hospital conducted a study which showed that 64 per cent of women who had given birth to their babies under general anaesthetic had neck and shoulder pains afterwards.

In the first few days after delivery

Even after your baby is born, you continue to be more vulnerable to back strain because your ligaments remain softened by the hormones of pregnancy for up to five months. One of these (relaxin), once thought to disappear soon after childbirth, may continue being produced for some while according to recent work by Dr Mark Johnson at the Chelsea & Westminster Hospital. Softer ligaments mean the bones and joints they are attached to cannot be held in place so well.

Common risk factors during the first few hours and days after the birth include:

- Breast- or bottle-feeding your baby without enough back support. You can be sitting in this position for hours every day so it is vital to be comfortable.

- Changing nappies, bathing or dressing the baby at an uncomfortable height for your back.

- Exhaustion: due to a tiring labour – or the lack of sleep that nearly all new babies bring.

- Lying down to rest so that your vulnerable back is strained or twisted in some way, or simply not supported well enough.

- Walking in a tentative, stooping shuffle, often with your head forward and shoulders tensed or hunched, because of sore perineal stitches which make walking painful. This can cause increased shoulder, neck and back tension until you can walk more freely. Massage, warm baths and other measures which encourage rapid perineal healing (see pp. 227–9) all help, as can mild pain relief.

- Neck and shoulder pain is more common after a general anaesthetic. Gentle massage, stretches and hot pads or hot baths can help, as can ordinary painkillers.

- Blinding, migraine-like headaches leading to considerable neck and shoulder tension for 24 to 48 hours after an epidural. Though they usually pass within a day or so they can make any movement, including breastfeeding, almost impossible while they last. Such headaches are not usual, but can be caused by a dural puncture (see p. 83).

After the first weeks

It is common to develop back trouble, even when you had none before, three or four months after delivery. Ligaments still soft from pregnancy will be kept soft if you are breastfeeding and this will make them vulnerable to the additional strains your back is being put under.

Potential culprits include:

- Buggy or pram handles at wrong height
- Changing, bathing and dressing babies at an awkward height for your back
- The position you sit in when you are feeding your baby, whether by breast or bottle
- Carrying babies, and maybe a jealous toddler too, for long periods (eg on your hip or in a sling while walking or cooking or doing housework)
- Using a back-damaging lifting technique. You will be doing a lot of lifting of the baby (especially if it is in a carry cot or a Moses basket) or other children you already have. Peak times for damaging your back include lifting babies/toddlers in and out of their cots, car seats and high chairs.

This is why it is very important to do the ante- and postnatal exercises which your midwife or hospital physiotherapist suggests, though it may feel like just one more thing you have to try and find time for, at first. Most maternity units will either make sure that one of the hospital physiotherapists comes round to see you to explain these before you leave, or at least give you a leaflet explaining how to do them. If they do neither, either ask to see the physiotherapist, or contact one of the childbirth or physiotherapy organizations (see **Resources**) for leaflets on postnatal exercise when you get home.

TREATMENT

It may be very helpful to go and see an osteopath or chiropractor who has a special interest in postnatal back care (many do – please see **Resources**) to have any joints or vertebrae which have become twisted out of alignment gently put right again.

In fact, it's a good idea, in the interests of catching any problems before they have the chance to develop, to go and have a back check-up at the six weeks after delivery mark, in the same way as you would go for a postnatal check-up with your doctor.

SELF-HELP MEASURES

- Attention to posture when sitting; have plenty of cushions and support at your back
- Try breastfeeding in a rocking chair or with your feet up on a footstool
- Make sure your pram handles are at the right height
- Lift with care so as not to strain your back
- Stand tall
- Do exercises to strengthen the muscles supporting the back
- Try yoga-based stretching exercises.

Please see pp. 268–9 for some of the most popular postnatal exercises. (See also pelvic floor exercises pp. 286–9; these may not help your back but are vital to prevent incontinence, prolapses and to help regain vaginal tone after delivery.)

Unfortunately, there is not enough room in this book to show in detail all the postnatal exercises you might be given through the different stages of recovery. Some you can begin the day after you have had your baby (such as foot flexing and gentle pelvic rocking). Others (pelvic lifts and sit ups) should not be tried until at least three months later, and only then if you have already been practising the gentler moves, or you could hurt yourself. See **Resources** for details of where to get the most helpful leaflets and books on postnatal exercises.

If you exercise regularly for the first few months after you have had your baby it will help your figure to return to normal faster, stop you developing back pain, and help prevent pelvic problems like urinary incontinence which affect about one in three new mothers.

Posture

Posture is the way you hold your body whether you are sitting, standing, walking, pushing.

Correct any changes in the way you do these things which may have developed gradually while you were pregnant without you even noticing them.

1. Standing position: You will be doing a lot of standing with young babies – rocking them, holding them on a hip or over your shoulder, cooking, telephoning and washing up holding them. Some are far more reluctant to be put down than others and may scream with astonishing staying power until you pick them up again.

These babies are not always happy to be just held while their mother sits down either. They often prefer to be walked around as well as held, and will renew their shouts until you do. Their mothers, in the interests of a quieter life, may find they are constantly on their feet if the baby is very demanding (American paediatricians and baby gurus William and Martha Sears call these 'High Need Babies'), has colic, or is unwell. If you have a baby like this it is especially important to:

A   *Keep reminding yourself that this phase will probably not last long*.

Usually by the time the babies can sit in bouncing swings (about four months) or use baby walkers (from six months) they will be so happy with their own new mobility that they will no longer demand you carry them about all day – just some of it. If they suffer from colic (which usually comes on in the evening for a few hours but may last on and off all day), they will usually grow out of this within 3 months. If your baby cries excessively, try contacting Cry-Sis, an organization which supports and counsels mothers whose babies cry a great deal or have colic; they can offer many practical and helpful suggestions (see **Resources**).

B   *Develop a good standing posture to protect your back:*

(i)   Stand in front of a long mirror and look at yourself sideways. Drop and relax your shoulders so your arms are hanging loosely and comfortably.

(ii) Stand up as tall as you can. Imagine a fine golden cord running through the middle of your body and out of the top of your head, pulling you upwards.

(iii) Tuck your buttocks in, then pull in your abdominals (your pubic bone should move forwards and upwards).

(iv) Move your feet about 12 inches apart.

(v)   Breathe slowly and deeply.

Feel your way mentally around the new way you are standing, notice how all the different muscles are working to hold you in this position, and how comfortable it feels. Deliberately stand tall at every possible opportunity.

Avoid wearing high heels. Go for trainers or shoes with a two and a half inch heel which will not put a strain on your back.

2. Feeding position: Draw your baby in towards you, whether you are breastfeeding or using a bottle, rather than leaning over to reach them. Sit well back in your chair, lower back well supported. It helps to place the baby on a pillow on your lap so it is raised up, and to put a stool, pile of phone directories, even the rung of a chair under your feet.

3. Working position for cooking, washing up, etc: Put one foot on the bottom shelf of an open cupboard just below where you are working, perhaps the cupboard under the sink when you are washing up, or on a pile of two or three phone directories kept in the kitchen for this purpose.

Rather than bending down, squat down with a straight back when doing 'low-level' jobs like making the bed, changing and dressing a toddler, sweeping something up with a dustpan and brush.

If at all possible, get someone else to do the vacuuming for the first few weeks as this can be a major strain on a vulnerable back. Be prepared to let floors get dirtier than usual for a while. Or, if you cannot avoid doing the vacuuming, move your weight to and fro over your front leg, keeping your back straight and avoiding making any twisting movements when you are bending forwards.

4. Changing your baby: Have a changing mat either:

(a) High enough so you do not have to bend over it. The baby should be lying level with the underneath of your breasts for the first few months, until it learns to roll over.

(b) Low down, at kneeling height, so you can change and wash them on your knees. In hospital, the only place is the bed – but this raises up and down so put it at a comfortable height (or get someone else to do it).

When you kneel, do not do so on both knees, as this is bad for your back too. Instead, sit back on either heel with the other knee bent forwards and the foot flat on the floor, pulling your baby as close to you as possible between your legs.

6. Lifting or carrying your baby and toddler: Be very careful when lifting them in and out of the car. The action of leaning forward, lifting the child's weight (plus carrycot or car cradle) and then twisting and lifting to bring them out of the car is a classic way for new mothers to injure their backs.

If someone else is around, ask them to do it. If not, squat down slightly to lift a toddler. For a baby in a car cradle with a handle or carrycot:

- sit sideways next to it with the car door open and slide it on to your lap
- swing both legs out of the car together
- hold on to the carrycot with one hand, using the free hand to hold on to the car door and help raise yourself slightly off the seat
- now release the car door and transfer your hand to support the baby's carrier while at the same time rising up off the seat using the buttock/leg muscles rather than the back muscles, keeping your back straight.

This is not nearly as complicated as it sounds. Try it out just once with an empty carrycot or baby basket, and you will find it is only three smooth movements.

When lifting a toddler or heavy bucket of soggy nappies pull your stomach muscles *in*, tuck your buttocks *under* and clench your pelvic-floor muscles. Then, keeping your spine straight, bend at the knees (squat right down if you need to) and bring the weight close in to your body. Using your *thigh* muscles, slowly stand up.

When carrying a baby along in a carrycot or basket, have the baby's head nearest to you.

Slings

Carrying a baby in a sling on your front or back places the least strain on your back. However, when younger people fall they usually tend to do so forwards (old people tend to slip backwards) so perhaps carrying a baby on your back might be safest.

Back slings are very comfortable but it can be a bit difficult to put a very young, floppy baby in one by yourself. It becomes easier as they gain more control over their necks and upper backs, at the age of three to four months.

If you are later using a *hip sling*, alternate the side it is on, so that both hips spend equal amounts of time bearing the baby's weight. Switch to carrying your baby on your back in a sling or African-style broad fabric sash after they reach about six months old, as then they will have become too heavy to carry for long on your hip without putting potentially damaging strain on your back.

Place pads of material – rolled up soft tea towels or a towelling nappy folded into a protective pad will do fine – under each of the sling straps as they press into your shoulders or you may develop very sore shoulder muscles, which can soon translate into generalized acute, painful neck and upper back tension.

If you do develop muscle spasms in your shoulders from this, they can be severe enough to make the shoulder muscles running from the top of your arm to your neck feel as hard as blocks of wood. Stop using the sling for a while. If the tension and pain remain entrenched, acupuncture or acupressure with massage beforehand is a good way of dispersing it rapidly (see **Resources**).

7. Bathing your baby: Even if you use a high enough surface not to need to bend over, you still have to pick up the bath and carry it to a sink or bath to empty the water out afterwards. This can be both heavy and awkward.

Some families get around this problem by using a large, very clean washing up bowl which fits into the (clean) sink in their (warm) kitchen. As long as the sink is at the right height, this puts the bathing baby at a good height for your back. It also means you do not have to lift and carry a small but heavy bath of water anywhere afterwards to empty it.

Alternatively, you might consider choosing a baby bath with a drainage plug in it, put it in the bath and fill it from the shower. Kneel next to it on *one* knee, keeping the other bent to maintain a straight back, and bath your baby. Then just let the water drain out through the plug afterwards. If you kneel on two knees it will still hurt your back.

Another good, safe, non-slip way of bathing your baby in an adult-sized bath is to get a large sponge which has a cut-out baby shape in the middle (available from most good department stores, or large baby equipment shops), and lay the baby on this. The warm water in the bath should come only part of the way up their body. Then kneel by the side of the bath as described above, and gently squeeze water from a flannel over them or splash the warm water softly over the baby's body.

A method which many babies enjoy enormously and which is one of the least troublesome ways to give them a bath, especially if they seem a little nervous of water or dislike their own small bath, is to get a rubber bath mat so you do not slip, run a warm (slightly above tepid) bath that is deep enough for both you and your baby and get in with them, letting them lie back, head slightly raised out of the water, on your chest, feet pointing downwards, so they float lightly on your breasts and stomach. Or lie them in the same place on their fronts, head to one side.

Be especially careful not to slip getting in and out, holding the baby close against you and moving slowly. It may be a good idea to have your partner in the room the first few times if you can, until you become used to doing this. Have a towel hanging ready next to the tub to wrap the two of you in.

8. Lying down: If your bed is very soft, slide a board under the mattress. Or put the mattress on the floor.

Ideally, lie on your front, as it is very helpful for relieving backache. Put one or two pillows under your waist to raise your pelvis and flatten your back. Place a couple more under your head and shoulders if you have swollen tender breasts.

If you like lying on your back, it may be comfortable to put a pillow under your knees or thighs. If you prefer to lie on your side, put one pillow against the small of your back and another between the knees.

When you get out of bed, do not twist or turn with your knees apart. Instead:

(i) Tighten your abdominal muscles

(ii) Bend your knees

(iii) Roll onto your side

(iv) Push yourself up into a sitting position with your arms

(v)   Keeping your knees together, swing both legs off the edge of the bed.

Do the reverse when getting back into bed.

Back support

Additional support is unlikely to weaken your back provided you are doing back-strengthening exercises, and it can make you feel far more comfortable in the first few weeks after birth.

A panty girdle may seem old-fashioned, but it will provide gentle back and abdominal support. It also has the added advantage of making you look deceptively flatter and firmer in front, as if you have suddenly regained your figure. Get your partner or a friend to drive you to a good local department store where there are trained fitters (such as the bra department of a John Lewis store). It's best to have professional help available to choose the best type and size for you.

A home-made binder sash is a traditional equivalent of the panty girdle, still worn in some parts of the world. They can be made of leather, woven grass, or material; some are wide, others simply consist of a piece of cord which is tightened a little every day. The binders may be used for a few days or in some cases three or four months after the birth, and in many societies they are worn with pride as an honourable sign that the woman is a new mother. Modern Japanese women still use a sash called a *hara-obi* from the middle of their pregnancies until about three weeks after they have had their babies. Mothers who wear them say it makes them feel more comfortable, especially if they are walking out and about or have to stand for long periods.

Birth educator and anthropologist Sheila Kitzinger suggests you make your own sash using a long crepe bandage 15–20cm wide, and 4.5m long. As it needs to go around you three times, you can make two or three binders out of this one piece of cloth. Wind it firmly around your lower abdomen and the small of your back, but not so tightly it interrupts circulation. You should, she says, feel 'neatly packaged but not constricted'.

Relieving low backache

The following stretches and exercises can help relieve low backache:

1 The Cat Arch
  - Kneel on all fours.
  - Blow all the air in your lungs out, and arch your back like a cat by tucking in your buttock and abdominal muscles.
  - Hold for four counts then relax until your back is flat again.
  - Repeat ten times, increasing to twenty. This exercise not only helps aching backs but strengthens your buttock and abdominal muscles.

2. Rocking Twists
  - Lie on your back on the floor.
  - Bend your left leg, and hook your toes under the right side of your calf, rolling your knee towards the right.
  - Place your right arm right across your body, so that the hand holds your left hip.
  - Rock from side to side gently, then roll back to the starting position again.

3. The Frog Stretch (see fig. 15)
  - Kneel on the floor and spread your knees as wide as you comfortably can.
  - Stretch gently upwards, reaching up as far as you can.
  - Lower your arms together in front of you: keeping them straight, stretch them right out in front of you as they come down towards the floor.
  - Keeping your back straight, push the palms flat against the floor and slide them along in front of you until you are reaching forwards as far as you can comfortably go.
  - It may be comfortable to just rest your forearms on the floor, or you may be able to stretch out fully. Rest in whichever position you can reach for a minute or two, then come back up slowly.

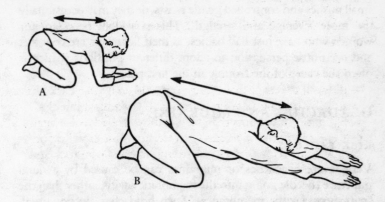

The Frog Stretch. This is very helpful if you have backache while you are pregnant, or at any stage after you have had your baby.

Swimming may well help too, if you can get a chance to do it at least once or twice a week.

PERSISTENT BACK PROBLEMS

If your problems persist for more than a few weeks, and neither gentle stretching nor exercises seem to help, go and see a registered osteopath or chiropractor who has a special interest in helping women with postnatal back problems. Many do, and some offer pregnancy check-ups of women's backs and general posture (plus a standard postnatal one too) as a preventative measure to help stop pregnancy-related back problems occurring in the first place (see **Resources** for advice on finding a therapist and for details of clinics offering treatment for reduced fees).

You may well start to feel relief from the first session. Unless there is a serious problem, you will probably need between two and six sessions altogether.

Chiropractors and osteopaths have slightly different techniques, but both use gentle manipulation of the spine and sometimes adjoining limbs to realign any joints or bones which have become badly positioned. They may do this with gentle pressure, small pushes and controlled gentle twists, or they may occasionally use more leverage and strength. This is seldom necessary for women who have just had babies, as their ligaments are very soft and need little persuasion to adopt different positions (which is often the cause of the trouble in the first place).

HEADACHES AND MIGRAINE

RISK FACTORS

Very severe headaches or migraines can be caused by a dural puncture (needle going into the membrane cavity, rather than the space between the membranes). Such headaches are not usual. Though they should pass within 24–48 hours they can make any movement, including breastfeeding, almost impossible while they last.

SELF-HELP MEASURES

- Try lying still, keeping light and movement to a minimum, eyes shut.
- Ask for any strong pain relief the staff can recommend (make sure the medication would not linger in your system and affect any later breastfeeding).
- Ask for visitors to be kept away, and for plenty of practical help with your baby.
- Ask if there is a single NHS room free (often called an 'amenity room'); ask if you can be moved to it tell the migraine subsides. These rooms will be slightly off the main ward.

Difficulties Which May Need Surgery to Put Them Right

Many problems which cause pain and discomfort after childbirth will settle down within a couple of weeks, and most within three months. However, for about 1 in every 100 women, childbirth may cause some structural damage to the pelvic area which will not resolve itself within six to twelve months and will therefore need to be corrected with surgery.

Unfortunately only a small proportion of the women who need this type of help ever get it.

HOW COMMON ARE THESE PROBLEMS?

There are no reliable figures. Professor Michael Chapman, former head of Obstetrics & Gynaecology at Guy's Hospital in London, estimates that 10 per cent of women experience pain or discomfort for any of the reasons listed below (the most common being a painful episiotomy site) for at least three to six months. Occasionally, this can mean intercourse will be painful for up to three years.

The most frequent problems are:

- An episiotomy site (or a labial tear) which has not healed properly is probably the most common problem. The area may be uncomfortable even when touched firmly at medical examinations, and may cause acute pain if you try to have sexual intercourse.

- Haematomas and haemorrhoids which refuse to heal. The former can be sore to touch, the latter may itch and cause discomfort and pain when you empty your bowels.

- A prolapse, either of the womb, vagina, cervix or rectum. This can cause a dragging, aching feeling, constant discomfort and backache.

- Over-stretching of the labial tissues or vagina, possibly due to a very rapid delivery where there was not enough time to stretch gently and gradually. This can cause sexual difficulties (either physical or perceived). It can also be very uncomfortable, because if the labia have been pulled out of shape, they can no longer fit closely and comfortably together to protect the delicate mucus membranes which line their inner surfaces and this can result in rubbing and friction there. It also increases the likelihood of infections such as thrush and vaginitis developing, which can be both itchy and painful.

Most of these problems do clear up with time, usually within six months of having given birth. If you do experience any of them, mention them at your six-week check-up so the extent of the problem can be assessed. Self-help measures may be very useful for some types of problems. A mild prolapse, for instance, could resolve with a programme of pelvic floor exercises. Others, like badly healed tears or episiotomies, would need surgical repair.

EPISIOTOMY AND TEAR SITES

WHAT IS IT?

An episiotomy is a sterile scissor cut made in your perineum, the muscular area between your vagina and anus. It would usually be carried out in the final stage of labour to create more room for your baby's head to get past, to help prevent major tearing and damage to the mother's perineal area, and to speed up the delivery. A tear is when the skin, or skin and some of the soft tissue below it, gives way naturally along the line of least resistance while the mother is pushing her baby out.

The cut would be made during a contraction, when the baby's head is stretching the perineum as far as it can go. Although the area is generally already numbed by this extreme stretching, the hospital will probably give a local anaesthetic too. You can specifically ask for one if there is enough time for it to be given and to take effect.

An episiotomy cut can heal rapidly, providing it has been properly repaired, as the blood supply to this area is very rich. While it is healing it may remain tender, or downright painful, for some time but there is a great deal which can be done to alleviate any trouble it may cause.

According to the Royal College of Obstetricians, episiotomies are carried out in about 50 per cent of all births in the UK, and are more often performed for first births than subsequent ones. Two thirds of first-time mothers and a third of mothers who have had babies before will have this surgery. Perineal tears are more common in first-time mothers too.

Whether episiotomies are done too readily and too often is a subject of an ongoing and very heated debate between natural birth groups/progressive obstetricians/midwives and the more mainstream clinical establishment. As Beverley Beech, chairwoman of the Association for Improvements in the Maternity Services puts it, in the 1940s if a woman needed an episiotomy her midwife would be 'on the carpet and called upon to explain herself'.

There are varying degrees of tears or cuts to the perineum which can occur as the woman reaches the late pushing stage of her labour:

First-degree. These just affect the skin of the perineum or the labia. If they are stitched promptly and properly they rarely cause any problems at all, and tend to heal within only two or three days. In many cases they do not need any stitching at all.

Second-degree. These go through the muscle as well as the skin.

Again, if stitched properly (and promptly – within about half an hour) they rarely cause problems. Usually the area stops being sore after 10 to 14 days. An episiotomy is generally equivalent to a second-degree tear.

Third-degree. These extend from the vaginal and perineal tissues into the rectum. They may be an extension of an episiotomy, if the mother has had an especially difficult birth with a big baby. Third-degree tears heal well if they have been promptly sewn up by an experienced member of staff after the baby is born. It is very important that an expert does the stitches, otherwise the woman may experience bowel incontinence.

If the cut or tear is a small one it may well heal on its own without stitching. Because the area is sore, women tend to keep their legs fairly close together and move carefully so as not to stretch and put any tension on the perineum at all, which also encourages healing. In many parts of Australia, small cuts and tears are not routinely sutured unless the mother especially wishes it; instead they are kept very clean and dry, and left to heal on their own. There are two ways to do an episiotomy cut:

(a)   Medio lateral – off to the side.
(b)   Midline – in a straight line from the fourchette down towards the anus.

Some doctors say the latter heal best, and in Canada and North America the medio lateral type is seldom done. In Britain, most midwives and obstetricians have been taught to do the former, saying that with midline cuts there can be a danger of the incision tearing down into the anal area too.

A neat episiotomy is easier to sew up than an uneven tear, but second-degree tears (ie those involving only skin and muscle), which are the most common variety, tend to heal more easily and rapidly than a cut. However, several large tears occurring along several different lines of least resistance as the baby's head is born are harder to repair well than a single large cut.

There is also a great difference between a *routine* episiotomy, done perhaps because of rigid hospital policy limiting how long a woman may remain in the second stage of labour, and a *necessary* one that is carried out because of a labour complication. Typical complications leading to a necessary episiotomy include:

- The baby being in a difficult position for delivery.
- Delivery of a premature baby whose head is softer than that of a full term infant. The episiotomy will reduce the pressure of the mother's vagina against the baby's skull.
- A baby who is too large to pass comfortably down and out of the vaginal canal.
- The delivery stage has been going on for such a long time that both mother and baby are becoming exhausted.
- Assisted delivery with forceps or vacuum extraction.

'My husband and me really wanted to make love again as I had been right off sex for the last half of my pregnancy with Carl. By six weeks the stitches had healed up into a nice, neat scar so we thought it would be fine. It wasn't. And we had to take things very slowly and gently for months because though a scar may not hurt if you press it yourself, the rubbing of intercourse is something else. You do begin to wonder whether it will ever be the same again down below.'

'I had an episiotomy three years ago and there are still certain sexual positions which put pressure on that area which are no longer comfortable for me.'

HOW LONG DOES IT TAKE TO HEAL?

About three-quarters of women will no longer be sore in this area after 10 days, but for 8–10 per cent the discomfort may persist for three months. Some women are uncomfortable for much longer than this, and may experience sexual difficulties as a result.

However, once the cut or tear has been properly stitched, there is a great deal that both you and any medical staff can do to encourage the area to heal quickly. Back in the 1920s, maternity units used to tie new mothers' knees together and keep them in bed thinking this helped the perineum to heal better. Now the range of treatments available includes crushed-ice packs, herbal baths, local anaesthetics and ultrasound.

> 'I don't know what all the fuss was about. My stitches healed fine and weren't really a problem after a couple of weeks.'
>
> 'They were OK until they got infected and then they really hurt.'
>
> 'I felt like I was sitting on thorns. It turned out that the stitches had been done too tight.'
>
> 'I never remember I've had one now – there are no problems at all.'

SYMPTOMS

Symptoms of an episiotomy or tear which has not healed properly can include:

- Pain, ranging from the area being slightly sensitive to touch, to it being extremely painful to touch.

- Itching, especially if the scar has healed in a lumpy (keloid) fashion.

- Feeling as if your vagina is too small, or that there is a constant slight pulling and over tightness of the skin. This is likely to be because when the episiotomy site was stitched up it was done tightly. It tends to happen when there is no room left for the tissue swelling which always follows injury (and perineal tissues can swell substantially).

Your stitches should be feeling considerably better within a week or so. If they are not, speak to your GP or midwife and ensure they look into the reason for this so something can be done about it. There are several potential causes, including infection which can be swiftly treated with antibiotics, or that the stitches have been done tightly in which case they can be removed.

SELF-HELP MEASURES

Lying on your front is an excellent way of relieving the pain of episiotomy and tear repair stitches, piles and backache. Put one or two pillows under your waist so your pelvis is raised and your back flattened comfortably. An extra pillow or two under your front or shoulders is helpful to protect your breasts.

It may help to sit on a child's plastic swimming ring, or a foam ring of the sort which used to be used in elderly people's wards, to reduce pressure on your stitches while they are healing. The foam rings are no longer available in some NHS maternity wards, as they are thought to prevent blood returning to the heart by compressing the major veins in the legs if used for long periods, but that need not stop women buying their own (see **Resources**).

Cushioned seating rings can be especially useful if you are trying to breastfeed for the first time, as it is considerably easier in the beginning to get your baby latched onto your breast in the right position while you are sitting down rather than lying down. The latter is very comfortable once you have both got the hang of it, but it can be difficult in the first day or so to get the baby at exactly the right level to suck effectively. If you are in hospital, keep asking the midwives and nurses for help with this until you find it easier. You will quickly feel comfortable in this relaxing feeding position with some help at the right time.

'I could not sit in one position for long for about two weeks. Me and my children's swimming ring became inseparable. And for another four weeks it was still tender for sitting for long periods so I carried a soft cushion about. It even went with me to the cinema.'

'The warm baths and herb stuff were bliss – I really think they helped. I now take a bottle of made-up herbal mix with me as a present to all my friends who have just had babies. They are a bit surprised at first, but the last three all told me my bottle of muddy-green liquid was much more use than another bunch of flowers.'

The following can also be very helpful and soothing:

- Crushed-ice packs and cooling sprays, or soothing baths with essential oil, salt or herbal infusions added (see pp. 227–9 above).

- Soothing cold compresses. Wet half a dozen men's handkerchiefs, lay plastic layers between them (cut-up supermarket bags will do), then freeze the cotton and plastic sandwich in the fridge freezer compartment. Use them one at a time, twisted into a slim, flexible, and very cold pad, on the episiotomy site.

- Pour water over your vulva when you urinate (see p. 228). Keep the area very clean to help avoid infection. Wipe or pat dry from front to back after passing water or emptying your bowels.

- Keep the stitches as dry as possible between cooling, soothing treatments as soggy stitches become more easily infected.

- After baths, showers, urinating while pouring water over, etc some women use a hair dryer on a cool setting rather than a potentially abrasive and less than sterile towel or loo paper. The only problem with this is that hair dryers can harbour germs best not blown over a healing wound. A potential alternative is to have an electric light bulb shone over your perineum to dry the area with radiating heat instead of a stream of hot air. Try removing the shade of a lamp which you can pick up and move about; an Angle-poise lamp would be ideal. If you are drying your stitches manually, pat dry with soft tissue, or keep a separate clean towel for your genital area.

- Sanitary pads: you will need to wear these for several days to protect your pants from lochia discharge (the blood which comes from your womb as the area your placenta was attached to heals). It diminishes steadily, disappearing altogether between two to six weeks with great variation from one woman to another. Change sanitary pads regularly.

Though the newer slimline pads can be ideal for ordinary menstrual periods, if you are sore around the genital area and have healing tears or stitches, it is the old-fashioned, large, soft cottonwool and loose lint type that offer the most comfort. Look for the packets marked 'Night Size' or 'Maternity Pad'. One of the only brands still offering this type of towel are Dr Whites.

- KY Jelly: although stitches heal better when kept dry, according to Caroline Flint (President of the Royal College of Midwives and a practising independent midwife), if your stitches are very sore indeed, some KY jelly on a clean sanitary pad can be very soothing.
- Witch-hazel soaked pads, applied directly on to the perineum, may help to soothe and cool swollen or inflamed tissue. Some midwives say that witch hazel and glycerine together are even more helpful.

TREATMENTS

The following can be helpful for sore stitches, whether they are the result of an episiotomy cut or a natural tear. Though there is no conclusive evidence that any of them will help every woman, there are many reports saying they have all helped some, so they are worth trying:

- Spray Epifoam, a mildly anaesthetizing foam, on the area. It contains a mild steroid and anaesthetic, and the hospital or your GP can prescribe this for you.
- Lignocaine gel, an anaesthetic gel which the hospital can also give you. Also available in spray form.
- Tincture of the homeopathic remedy Hyper cal: a few drops on a soft sanitary pad is thought to help reduce soreness, encourage cooling and aid the healing process.

- Paracetamol can be useful for mild perineal pain. Or if this does not help, try a non-steroidal anti-inflammatory drug like aspirin. However, strong painkillers which contain a good deal of codeine are not so suitable. They can encourage constipation, and straining to empty your bowels is the last thing you need if you have perineal stitches – many women are constipated for a few days after giving birth anyway.

- Ultrasound and pulsed electromagnetic energy, commonly used for treating many types of sports injury, are thought to help reduce swelling by increasing the permeability of cell walls so fluid can flow back into them, as well as out to the spaces between the cells. Pulsed electromagnetic energy is thought to help heal damaged tissues by restoring the electrical balance of damaged cells.

   There is conflicting evidence as to whether these help or not. Nevertheless, most maternity units offer the treatments. They need to be done by a physiotherapist, and it can be given through a sanitary towel.

NOTE: Steroids may be added to some local anaesthetic gels and sprays.

SURGERY

Occasionally, if the stitching of the tear or episiotomy has not been done by someone who was competently trained, poor suturing techniques may cause the underlying muscles to distort so the labia, perineum and vaginal lining are badly aligned.

Both doctors and midwives who are learning how to do suturing should *always* be carefully supervised. Some of the former may never have done this type of stitching before. It requires skill, and different techniques from the more straightforward ones employed when a cut on the arm or leg is sewn up in the Accident & Emergency department.

Another reason for poor healing of cuts or tears around the vagina, perineum and labia is that the edges have not been brought together so they lie flush with each other, says Professor

Chapman. Instead they have overlapped or shelved – especially likely if the tear is a jagged one which happened naturally rather than a clean cut done by the obstetrician or midwife as an episiotomy.

Sometimes granulation and fibrosis occur over the stitched area, preventing it from healing flat. These tissue overgrowths may also develop tiny new blood vessels to supply them, and so develop into living lumps, which means the scar will remain raised. This is more prone to happen to a small or large wound if the area is not kept dry, and it is difficult to keep a vagina moisture-free.

If the scar has healed badly and is still painful, it may need to be recut along its original site and sewn up once more, carefully and evenly. This needs to be done under general anaesthetic and will be as sore as it was originally for a few weeks, but then should gradually begin to improve until it causes no discomfort at all.

You may need to do all the things you did to soothe the pain it caused after you had just given birth. Take regular herbal or saline baths, use crushed-ice packs on the area, sit on a child's swimming ring, and keep the stitches dry.

Surgery may also be necessary if a small nerve has been trapped when the episiotomy repair was done. This is unusual, though it does occasionally happen, and can be difficult to detect as there is nothing to actually see even if a woman is examined carefully. But the area can be exceptionally painful, making intercourse impossible even after any incisions have healed perfectly months ago.

HAEMATOMAS

WHAT ARE THEY?

Haematomas are small sacs filled with clotted blood. They feel like small lumps underneath the perineal skin, and can be very tender to touch.

RISK FACTORS

They develop as a result of strenuous pushing to help the baby out. They usually diminish within a week or two of the birth. Some, however, can go on to develop fibrosis and form scar tissue around themselves. They may also become infected.

TREATMENTS

One way to try and get rid of haematomas is to inject fluid into any fibrous tissue which has formed, to spread it out. This can be done under local anaesthetic. It is also possible for a surgeon to try stretching them manually to break down the fibrous tissues surrounding them. Again, this can be most uncomfortable and is best done under general anaesthetic. If neither of these works, they can be removed surgically. They can also be eradicated using cold treatment (freezing the area) under local anaesthetic.

HAEMORRHOIDS

WHAT ARE THEY?

Haemorrhoids are piles, which are produced by the enlargement of the blood-vessels in the wall of the anus. They can be very uncomfortable, especially if you are sitting for long periods.

SYMPTOMS

Apart from feeling small lumps in and around your rectum, you may experience:

- pain
- itchiness
- discomfort when you have a bowel movement passing across them
- bleeding when you have a bowel movement.

They can protrude from the wall of the anus, and will either return spontaneously or have to be pushed back in.

RISK FACTORS

Piles also develop as a result of strenuous pushing to help the baby out and should subside within a week or two of the birth. Some however never quite disappear, and may be made worse by subsequent pregnancies. If they refuse to subside on their own, they can be dealt with by minor surgery.

TREATMENT

A GP could prescribe a haemorrhoid-shrinking ointment for you. These often contain an anti-irritant agent to help soothe itching. If this is not helpful, they may need minor surgical treatment, possibly ligature, which involves tying off the individual haemorrhoids tightly under general anaesthesia so the excess fleshy protrusions wither away and fall off. This would not be done until three to six months after delivery.

PROLAPSE

WHAT IS IT ?

Damage to an organ or internal part of the body so it drops downwards from its usual position, usually because its supporting tissues have been damaged or weakened. Childbirth is a very common cause of prolapse.

There are several different types which can be caused by the stretch of late pregnancy and by labour. *They are not usually enough of a problem to need surgical repair for some years*. However, in some cases they may be sufficiently noticeable for you to have one or more of the symptoms listed below. Equally, you may notice nothing wrong at all.

SYMPTOMS

Prolapse of the womb

The symptoms are similar to a prolapse of the vagina, and can include:

(i)   In the case of a minor prolapse you may experience a very slight dragging feeling. If the problem is more severe, you will actually feel something bulging out at the top of your vagina, by the cervix.

(ii) A dragging ache around your lower abdomen.

(iii) Backache.

(iv) Fatigue.

Prolapse of the rectum or bladder

This is caused by damage to the tough, fibrous wall between the rectum or bladder and vagina. If you feel something bulging through into the back wall of the vagina when you have a full bowel and need to empty it, it is called a rectocele. When the bulge can be felt through the front wall of the vagina, that is the bladder when it is full, and the condition is called a cystocele. Symptoms, if you are aware of them, may include:

(i)   When you cough a slight bulge can be felt in the vagina on either the back or front wall as you slide your finger gently in there.

(ii) An aching or dragging feeling around your perineum, the muscular area dividing the entrance of your vagina from the entrance of your rectum.

Vaginal prolapse

This is caused by damage to the vagina so that it prolapses downwards, protruding slightly into the labial area.
Symptoms, if any, may include:

(i) A slight but continual sensation, described by women who have experienced it as 'a feeling of bagginess' or 'drooping' in the vagina.

(ii) You may find that you can pull it back up into position by doing a pelvic lift movement, and that wearing a tampon is uncomfortable because it drags at the already stretched vaginal tissue when it is removed.

(iii) You may find you are more prone to vaginal infections.

(iv) You may find the protrusion itself uncomfortable; it may be rubbed by tight pants and become sore. The fact that something is in the labial area which should not be there can itself feel uncomfortable. Even if it does not actually hurt, it simply does not feel right and the woman may be constantly aware of it.

(v) Feeling as if you need to pass water frequently.

(vi) You will be more prone to developing urinary infections like cystitis.

Prolapse of the cervix

This often drops down slightly from its usual position during pregnancy, and does not fully return after delivery.

Symptoms, if any, may include:

(i) A bulge about the size of a cherry at the top of your vagina.

(ii) You may also experience an aching, dragging feeling in your lower abdomen.

SELF-HELP MEASURES

Pelvic exercises

The pelvic floor is the sling of muscles which holds up all the internal abdominal organs, including the womb, bladder, intestines and rectum. Pelvic exercises are often the first line of treatment to try. With certain types of prolapses they can help you avoid the need for surgery at all. However, it is important to check with your gynaecologist or obstetrician first that the type of prolapse you have could benefit.

These exercises can also be useful if, on top of everything else, you are suffering from stress incontinence (finding it difficult to hold back when you either want to pass water or a bowel movement). One in three women are thought to have some degree of incontinence after childbirth, and the mechanical damage that a baby may cause while it is being born can lead to incontinence, or prolapses. This is because the pelvic floor takes the brunt of the force with which the baby descends. Because similar types of damage to the pelvic soft tissues and suspensory ligaments have similar effects, it also means that muscle exercises which can help incontinence can also benefit a mild prolapse.

You can do pelvic exercises by yourself at home, but they need to be done properly to be effective. It's not just a matter of clenching your bottom or squeezing your urine-stopping muscles as often as you can – so it helps if you have someone to show, or explain to you the right way to carry them out and help you with any difficulties you are having with them. There are specially trained continence nurses at some general hospitals and in the community, attached to larger GP practices, who can do this. There are also several good self-help organizations which have trained continence nurse counsellors who can advise you over the phone, such as Continence Line (see **Resources** for their address and phone number). They treat all calls in the strictest confidence and you do not even have to give your name if you do not want to.

Pelvic exercise options

Pelvic exercises can be done:

- Actively, as you would do stomach-flattening sit ups.
- They can be helped with electrical equipment at the hospital physiotherapy department. The equipment gives the muscles extra stimulus as you work them.

- You can use vaginal training weights and cones as internal exercise aids. Ask your physiotherapy department if you can borrow a set of these for home use – or where you can buy some for yourself.

Try to do these exercises as soon as possible. Even if you only do a few in the first few days very gingerly indeed it will improve the circulation to this area, which in itself can help promote healing. However, some women find it very difficult if not downright impossible to do pelvic lifts after giving birth because their perineum has been damaged by a tear or episiotomy. The area may also feel numb and refuse to respond to your efforts to mobilize it for a few days. If it really hurts, wait another couple of days until the area has healed a little further and you can use the muscles more easily. If you are still unable to flex your pelvic muscles even after the area has healed, tell your GP and ask to be referred to a specialist for help – these muscles need using, to avoid problems such as prolapse and incontinence.

To get the most out of pelvic floor exercises you will need to do them as many times a day as you can (at least three or four). It's also important that you locate the right muscles to exercise, which isn't always easy. There are three sets of muscles you need to find:

a   The sphincter muscle, which opens and shuts the neck of your bladder

b   The muscles which control your anus

c   The muscles which you use to squeeze and relax your vagina.

To find **a**, try stopping the flow of urine next time you pass water. The muscles you squeeze while trying to do that are the ones of your bladder sphincter.

To find **b**, pretend that you are desperate to empty your bowels (or wait until you really are) then make yourself hang on for a while longer. The muscles you are using now are the ones controlling your anus.

To find **c**, flex the muscles you usually use in your vagina to grip or squeeze your partner's penis when you are having intercourse. If you are not quite sure if you are flexing the right ones (as there are so many bands of muscle in the pelvic area and it is sometimes hard to separate the action of one from another set lying near them), slide a clean finger or tampon applicator into your vagina and then try squeezing that.

To do one full pelvic floor exercise, you need to squeeze each of these sets of muscles in turn: **a, b, c.** Hold each for a count of four and release, then tighten them all together and 'pull up' the whole lot at once so the entire sling of muscle across your pelvic floor lifts upwards. This is called the pelvic smile, because that is the shape the muscles are now making inside you.

Get into a slow, easy rhythm for doing this – saying something like: '**Front** (pee-stopping muscles) **Back** (bowel-stopping ones) **Middle** (vaginal muscles) **Pull up.**' Repeat perhaps four times a session at first, working up to twenty, thirty, forty or fifty times each exercise session. Do these sessions four or five times a day; more if you can.

Pelvic floor strengthening exercises may well be enough to solve the problem for you, but you do have to do them faithfully for weeks rather than days. If you keep a diary of how many you do and how often you leak or lose urine (even if it is only a drop or two), you will hopefully be able to look back over the weeks and see how much improvement you have made.

You may wish to ask your doctor if you can be referred to the local hospital's physiotherapy department so you can use their passive electronic machines to stimulate your pelvic muscles too, as well as doing the active exercises. These work on the same principal as Slendertone beauty machines and can substantially enhance your own exercise efforts. The electrical pads are attached to your abdominal area; they do not need to be used internally.

In the right circumstances, internal weight training using small vaginal cones of different weights can also be a helpful addition to a pelvic toning regime. You start, as with any pelvic weight training, with the lightest – and practise holding it inside your vagina like a tampon for an increasing amount of time, then go on to the next, slightly heavier weight. Some women even walk around the house with one in. The physiotherapy department may have them or you can buy some from mail order companies (please see **Resources**). Always check with your doctor or physiotherapist that they would be suitable for you before you begin using them.

. If despite all your efforts the exercises do not seem to have made much difference after three months, return to see your obstetrician and ask them to examine you again, and insist that they consider a surgical repair for you.

MEDICAL TREATMENT

If you have a prolapsed womb and it has not been improved by at least three months' worth of rigorous pelvic floor exercises or is too severe to be suitable for these, you will need surgery to correct it but may have to wait a few months for the operation.

In the meantime your GP or gynaecologist can fit a pessary which is placed at the top of the vagina. It is a circular ring of plastic which fits around the cervix, holding the womb upwards and back while allowing the round cervix to protrude through a hole in the middle, so any menstrual blood can flow out normally.

The traditional pessary shape is a sort of ring bent into a fat S; this is called the Hodge pessary but this is now seldom used. The more usual shape is a simple ring made of soft rubbery plastic about a centimetre thick. It needs to be fitted by a doctor who has experience of this type of device, and many GPs will refer you to a hospital outpatients department for this (family planning clinics are not equipped to do it either).

The ring stays in for between three and six months when it needs replacing, so it is very important that it fits well. To make sure of this, it comes in a variety of different sizes; tell your doctor if the fit is at all uncomfortable. It does protrude down into the vagina slightly and though you will probably not be able to feel it, your sexual partner will.

Watch out for signs of infection when you wear one (the main signs are bad-smelling discharge or itching) and if you have any report them straight away. Pessaries also cause a certain amount of vaginal inflammation which could turn into an ulcer because of constant pressure on the delicate tissues, so report any discomfort.

These rings will not relieve all the symptoms of a prolapse; they are simply a holding measure until you can have corrective surgery.

SURGERY

Surgery for any sort of prolapse involves a general anaesthetic and a stay in hospital of about a week. Just exactly what the surgeon does depends on what is wrong.

The basis of most treatments is to take a surgical tuck in whatever muscle or ligament has been overstretched. Basically this is done by cutting it, removing any excess tissue and sewing it back up again. Prolapse operations are successful in about 80 per cent of all cases. Pelvic tissue repair of this sort is usually quite strong, because where a tuck has been taken in muscle or somewhere like the thick, tough fibrous wall between rectum and vagina, a certain amount of fibrosis (overgrowth of tough fibrous tissue) would cover the area which had been stitched, reinforcing it further. However, in about half of all cases, the problem can return later.

Occasionally, if the prolapse of a womb is severe, a surgeon may suggest a hysterectomy for a woman who has completed her family.

In the first six to twelve months after you have had your baby, doctors may be unwilling to do any surgery at all, even though there is a problem. There are some clinical reasons for not doing such a repair too promptly, including:

- The fact that many structural postnatal problems, from a mild prolapse to a sore episiotomy site, can improve considerably on their own within six to twelve months.

- Prolapses do not usually happen until several years later following further pregnancies, the effect of the menopause, and general ageing, so it is unusual for younger women to need a prompt operation to repair one. The seeds of a prolapse may be sewn now – but it will not usually develop into a condition needing repair for some years. The best way to prevent one is to try and get into the habit of doing pelvic exercises several times a day – every day.

- After tissues are repaired they are left permanently weakened by the surgery and stitching so there is a good chance that the problem may recur (about fifty-fifty) around the time of the menopause. This is because the pelvic tissues lose elasticity and strength as their supply of oestrogen diminishes naturally, and if there is an existing weakened area it may well break down again (often not on the scar site but next to it), meaning a re-repair which will in its turn be even more of a weak link.

- If a woman wants more children and it is clear that her pelvic floor has been weakened so as to produce the beginnings of a prolapse there, she is advised to use temporary measures, such as a vaginal support ring pessary for a womb prolapse or vaginal prolapse, until she has completed her family – and then have the repair operation.

- If she has already had any type of repair, either of a stitches site or for pelvic floor damage, and it is feared that pregnancy and labour would damage it all over again, she would be advised to give birth to her subsequent babies by caesarean section.

Further, the weight of the developing baby and growing uterus could, together with the relaxant effect of pregnancy hormones upon all muscles and supporting ligaments, predispose her to another prolapse.

VAGINAL DISCOMFORT

If the vagina feels too tight after pregnancy it may be because of a sore scar area, a knob of tissue anywhere along the vagina's length which makes penetration difficult, or a vaginal/perineal repair done too tightly. The pain could also be caused by a nerve in the area that has been trapped by suturing.

SYMPTOMS

Some women will find it painful when the area is touched at all, others will only be aware of pain when they are trying to have intercourse.

FIRST LINE TREATMENT

Steroid creams may be useful. They are used for many types of scar such as lumpy keloid scars caused by severe acne, and may also help soothe any tenderness or itching.

SURGERY

However, poorly healed or badly done episiotomy/stitch sites usually need to be corrected surgically, perhaps to excise a lump of tissue, or to recut a lumpy scar along the vagina's length and sew it up again carefully. The general term for an operation to repair a vagina is colporrhaphy. This procedure might involve the slight loss of some vaginal tissue, as they are done in much the same way as a dressmaking dart is sewn into a piece of material to conceal a tear.

However, this is not always an easy operation to do, as it is possible for a surgeon who does not have sufficient experience to sew a vaginal repair up a little too well – with the result that the passage is too tight. This may also be a problem if they were trying to do a small tuck to correct slack vaginal tissues which had been permanently stretched by the baby's descent. The latter is not usual, but is more likely to happen with an extremely rapid delivery.

Even if the vaginal passage is now too small, it is usually possible to slowly expand it over a period of time by DIY internal massage with plain lubricant and your own finger or gentle, careful lovemaking. This process may take months and you will need a gentle, understanding partner to help make it work; or, in a relationship which has already been stressed, it may cause sexual difficulties by a continuation of the very problems that the surgery was meant to help resolve.

Aftercare for this type of operation includes all the things that help a post-delivery tear or cut to heal (see above, pp. 227–9).

DISCOMFORT OR PAIN AFTER A CAESAREAN SECTION

In Britain, 1 in 8 women have their babies by caesarean. Those who know no better may say: 'A caesarean? You did it the easy way then', or 'No labour pains – you were lucky, mine lasted 17 hours'. And even, if they have a sore episiotomy or tear: 'It's all right for you. At least you can sit down.'

In fact, the operation itself remains a major one even though it is very common and very safe. The necessary medical care immediately afterwards (together with a longer recovery time), may bring specific problems, though there are many strategies which can help enormously with post-caesarean difficulties.

The level of discomfort may depend not only on your own pain tolerance but also on the type of anaesthesia you had and whether you had your caesarean after a period of labour. Some women who have had more than one caesarean say they had different amounts of pain after each birth.

There is a wealth of practical and sympathetic advice available from the Caesarean Support Network (please see **Resources**) on the best way to do everything from getting out of bed painlessly to the feeding positions which will not put pressure on your scar site.

The following are some of the most important and helpful suggestions. But perhaps the best piece of advice is: *Accept all the help you are offered (providing it is not intrusive) and then ask for more when you find you need it – every time you need it.*

'I would not mind if I had my next baby this way, now I know what happens.'

'Once my epidural wore off it hurt every time I moved even a little. Even though I had painkillers four-hourly, I was needing more after only two and a half had gone by. They would not give them to me though.'

'My stomach felt badly bruised, my arm was sore where the drip had been in, I was sore down below from having a catheter there, the epidural site hurt and so did my breasts. I was a wreck.'

'I always had this idea that a caesarean was a sort of painless way to give birth, and I was glad to have one as I have always been very nervous of the idea of labour pains and pushing a baby out – I was sure I just couldn't do it as I am quite small and tight down there. But coming round after the anaesthetic I felt sick, groggy; it hurt me to move at all, I could barely hold my baby and I felt really incapacitated.'

'After the initial pain (especially on the first two or three days) I remember walking around more easily than some women who had had episiotomies.'

'I have had all three children by caesarean. I was a bit disappointed at the beginning, with my first – but I loved having the babies, and am not so bothered about how they arrive.'

IMMEDIATELY AFTER YOUR OPERATION

You will stay in hospital for 5 to 10 days afterwards, depending on how you are feeling and on the hospital's policy. After a spinal or epidural anaesthetic, you could theoretically go home within

24 hours if you had adequate pain relief and regular visits from your community midwife at home.

Day 1

The incision site, which will either be a bikini cut just above your pubic hair or, less usually, a vertical cut running down the centre of your abdomen, will be covered in a light dressing. There may be a drain, which will be left in place for a few hours to draw off any blood and fluid loss from your incision.

Help may include:

A   Strong pain relief:

   (i)   If you had an epidural this may well be left in place for a few hours and topped up slightly.

  (ii)   You may be given a push-button operated drug delivery system which you operate yourself and that feeds painkilling medication directly into your arm (see p. 95).

 (iii)   Painkilling injections or tablets. Check that they are drugs which will not affect your baby if you are planning to breastfeed.

 (iv)   Sleeping tablets at night for the first few days may be very helpful – ask the maternity ward staff. Check that the ones that you are offered will have no effect on the baby if you are breastfeeding.

B   Antibiotics: if there is any sign of post-operative infection, such as a raised temperature, you will be given antibiotics. These can, however, encourage itchy, sore vaginal thrush so you may need to take preventative measures against that (see below).

C   On the day of your operation and until 24 hours afterwards, restrict movement to cuddling your baby, sitting up slowly with help, and wriggling your toes or circling your feet while lying down to help get the circulation going. If you cough, laugh or sneeze this will make your newly stitched abdominal muscles tense, which will hurt. Lace your fingers together, and place your joined hands gently but firmly over the area to help support it. Ask to see the physiotherapist who will show you the best way to do this.

Caesarean sections and thrush

Women who have their babies by caesarean are usually given antibiotics routinely to avoid postoperative infection. These can make you more vulnerable to developing thrush, so consider asking for some preventative anti-thrush oral or pessary treatment while on the antibiotics.

You could also ask a friend or your partner to buy you some anti-thrush cream for vaginal use, and vaginal thrush pessaries, as both are now available over the counter in pharmacies. But tell them to make sure any cream they are sold is definitely for vaginal thrush. A recent report (*Drug & Therapeutics Bulletin*, 1994) found that most pharmacies sold women asking for anti-thrush fungicidal cream the wrong one, giving them the type used for athlete's foot instead.

Day 2

This may seem callous at the time because you will probably still be feeling very sore, but this is the day when you are strongly encouraged to get out of bed and try to walk around a little. Movement is vital to improve circulation (avoiding the formation of any blood clots) and help you recover faster.

Walking: Get a nurse or your partner to help you if this is the first time you have got up, as you may feel a bit dizzy and unsteady at first. Keep stopping for rests and gentle deep breaths, and do not overdo it on the first expedition out of bed. If you possibly can, try and avoid the Caesarean Shuffle – head down, dropped shoulders, hands supporting your abdomen and feeling worried your stitches may break open. They won't. And walking gets easier each time you do it, so walk as tall as you can.

Bathing: For the first day or two after your operation, you would find it difficult to get in and out of a bath, but a warm shower can be very soothing (your dressing may be removed before or afterwards). Check the water temperature before you get under, because you won't be able to jump away quickly if it is too hot. Arrange for someone to be there to help dry you and put you into your nightdress. Wear slip-on slippers as you don't have to bend over to put them on.

Getting out of bed: This may hurt too in the first few days. However it can help considerably to:

(i)   Ask for your bed to be lowered.

(ii)   Get out of bed slowly at your own pace.

(iii) Use deep breathing and relaxation techniques.

(iv) Take it in stages – many women find the following technique helpful:

- As you try and get up, put your chin on your chest, push your palms into the bed close to your sides, lifting your bottom a little to shuffle your body sideways.

- Repeat the movement until you reach the left side of your bed.

- Using both hands, lift your left leg from the knee to place your foot on the floor. Then your right leg.

Keep stopping for rests and gentle, deep breaths as often as you need to.

Sitting: Choose a high, upright chair, preferably one with arms. To sit down, it helps to put one leg behind the other, bending at the knees. To get up again, lean forward gently, put one leg behind the other and bend the knees.

Going to the toilet: Bend your knees to lower yourself down, holding on to any side rails.

You will be asked to try and pass water, and open your bowels within two to three days of your operation. Bowel movements may not be easy, as you will not have eaten or drunk anything for a while, and you may be worried too that your stitches will burst open if you strain to pass a bowel motion. It can help to:

(i)   Ask for a gentle laxative such as Lactulose the night before.

(ii)   Drink as many sips of water as you can, as often as you can and as soon as you can after your operation. Faeces absorb water, making them softer to pass.

(iii) Support your stitches gently and firmly with the flat of your hand as you push to empty your bowels.

(iv)   If your bowels have not opened by the fifth morning, some hospitals suggest a small enema of plain water to soften any waste matter in the rectum.

Wind: You may have wind pains a couple of days after your delivery. They may be mild or more severe. The Caesarean Support Network says that the following breathing exercise will help, and recommend that you start it as soon as possible after your baby is born, then repeat four times an hour.

(i)   Lace your fingers together and fold your joined hands over the incision to support it.

(ii)   Breathe in deeply and breathe out slowly.

(iii) Take another deep breath and hold it there for a count of five (ten, if you can manage it) then exhale slowly.

(iv)   Take a final deep breath and let it flow out.

It can also help to drink peppermint water, fennel tea, eat a few arrowroot biscuits or some extra strong mints. But avoid fizzy drinks like sparkling spring water or Lucozade.

Feeding your baby: If you are bottle-feeding, try and give the baby its feeds yourself and ask the nursing staff to help you find a comfortable position. If you are breastfeeding, you can do this as soon as you feel able after the delivery, even if you had a general anaesthetic and both you and the baby are still a little groggy (see p. 93).

Ask the nursing staff to help you find a comfortable position and to ensure that your baby is latching on to your breast properly. Do not worry if you feel awkward during the first feeds.

Most first-time mothers, and many new mothers of subsequent babies even when they have breastfed before, feel this way to begin with.

Whether you are breast- or bottle-feeding, you need to try and keep the baby's weight off your incision site. The following may be comfortable for you if you have a vertical scar:

- Sitting up with pillows across your stomach to absorb the pressure of the baby's small body.

- Lying on your side with your baby lying next to you. It can take a bit of practice at first to get the baby at the right 'height' to feed from your breast this way, but once you develop the knack of it, it is very comfortable – especially if you are feeling tired.

- Putting a pillow on the meal trolley which fits over your bed and placing the baby on this.

If you have a bikini scar:

- Tuck the baby under your arm, lying on a pillow, her head facing your breast or a bottle and her body under your arm.

- Placing your baby on a pillow on the meal tray as above.

- Sitting up with a pillow supporting you on either side, her head on one of those pillows and her feet on your thighs.

General comfort: If your pubic hair was shaved* rather than clipped very short for your operation it can be extremely itchy when it grows back. It helps to sprinkle the area with cooling zinc or baby talcum powder, and pat it in.

The pain or discomfort from the incision site may fade into itchiness and sensitivity, then cease to cause you any problems at all. Wear waist-high soft cotton pants if you have a bikini scar and larger, looser clothes without waistbands while you are healing.

---

* This is very seldom necessary, but some hospitals still insist on doing it routinely. If you are reading this section *before* you go in for a caesarean birth, let the staff know (perhaps as part of your birthplan) that you do not wish to be shaved.

Resources

BOOKS

The following may be both helpful – and interesting – to pregnant women thinking about the form of pain relief they would like. Some are about a particular method such as water, others look at what traditional societies do; some cover the mechanics of labour and others the issues surrounding the first few weeks and months after you have had your baby. If you cannot find any of them in a local bookshop, you can order them via your library if you give them the publisher's name and publication year.

The National Childbirth Book of Pregnancy, Birth and Parenthood ed. by Glynnis Tucker (Oxford University Press, 1992).

Who's Having Your Baby? by Beverely Beech (Camden Press, 1987). On women's rights in all aspects of childbirth.

Just Close Your Eyes . . . and Relax by Dr Les Brann (Thorsons, 1987). A book and tape of a self-hypnosis programme for childbirth.

Water Birth by Janet Balaskas and Yehudi Gordon (Thorsons, 1992). There is also a video showing three waterbirths plus interviews with the parents and midwives, available by mail order from the Active Birth Centre (see below).

The Caesarean Experience by Sarah Clement (Pandora Books, 1991).

The Unborn Child – How to Recognise and Overcome Perinatal Trauma by Roy Ridgeway (Wildwood House, 1987). Despite its daunting title this is not written for the medically qualified. It is a sympathetic and wide-ranging review of material about the sensibilities of the unborn baby – what it may remember, and how its birth might affect it in later life.

Breastfeeding Your Baby by Sheila Kitzinger (Dorling Kindersley, 1989) and *Getting Breastfeeding Right for You* by Mary Renfrew, Chloe Fisher and Suzanne Arms (Celestial Arts, Berkeley, California, 1990).

Exercising after Pregnancy by Barbara Whiteford and Margie Polden (Century Books, revised edition 1988). Sensible, easy to follow exercises from two obstetric physiotherapists. Many of them you can do with your baby. Designed to target the pelvic floor and back, to help avoid back pain, pelvic pain and continence problems postnatally.

Childbirth Wisdom – from the World's Oldest Societies by Judith Goldsmith (East West Health Books, 1990).

Birth Traditions and Modern Pregnancy Care by Jacqueline Vincent Priya (Element Books, 1992). The author runs the Birth Traditions Survival Bank in Malawi.

Alternative Medicine by Dr Andrew Stanway (Penguin, revised edition 1986) compact and succinct guide to all the different complementary therapies; see also *The Readers Digest Family Guide to Alternative Medicine* (Readers Digest Association, 1991).

Yoga for Pregnancy by Janet Balaskas (Element Books, 1994). Audio casette and booklet available from Active Birth Centre.

How to Survive Your Pregnancy by Geoffrey Chamberlain (Quadrant Press, revised ed. 1989).

LEAFLETS

A series of leaflets on many aspects of pregnancy and birth, including pain relief and caesarean section, are published by the Royal College of Obstetricians and Gynaecologists. Available at £1.50 each from the RCOG Bookshop, 78 Park Road, London NW1 4RG.

HELP GROUPS AND USEFUL SERVICES

When writing to any of the support groups listed below, please enclose a stamped addressed envelope. Many are run by unpaid volunteers and are constantly short of funds.

The Active Birth Centre/Movement, 55 Dartmouth Park Road, London NW5 (tel. 0171 267 3006). Runs one- to four-day courses nationwide on active childbirth techniques, contact above number for nearest one to you. They also supply extensive literature on the subject (including several books and a catalogue of products helpful in pregnancy and labour) and offer advice and support for women who want to try for a natural childbirth, water birth, or use water in their labour. They will hire out a range of portable birthing pools from around £90 to £140 for four weeks, and can let you know which private and NHS hospitals in your area have a water pool as part of their maternity facilities.

Ainsworth Homeopathic Pharmacy, 38 New Cavendish Street, London W1 (tel. 0171 935 5330). Offers good advice and a mail-order service.

Aromatherapy Organizations Council, (tel. 01455 615 466). Umbrella body for the major aromatherapy organizations, with a register of professionally qualified members. May also be able to advise on those who have a special interest in helping women during pregnancy and childbirth.

Association of Breastfeeding Mothers, Sydenham Green Health Centre, 26 Holmshaw Close, London SE26 (tel. 0181 778 4769). Has a national helpline offering telephone advice and support (and visits if distances permit) to help mothers with all aspects of breastfeeding difficulties including breast pain. Also runs some local support groups.

Association of Chartered Physiotherapists in Obstetrics and Gynaecology, c/o The Association of Chartered Physiotherapists, 14 Bedford Row, London WC1 (tel. 0171 242 1914). Will offer advice and information on exercises to correct postural and pelvic problems (especially back pain and incontinence) often associated with pregnancy and birth. Have some helpful leaflets too.

Association for the Improvement of Midwifery Services (AIMS), 21 Iver Lane, Buckinghamshire (tel. 01753 652781). AIMS offers information and advice on all aspects of your maternity options and rights. You can speak to its representatives over the phone; they respond rapidly to letters, and can send you their own leaflets and reports on a wide variety of issues concerning pregnancy and childbirth such as prenatal scanning, episiotomy, epidurals, and all your choices in childbirth.

Association for Medical and Dental Hypnosis, 42 Links Road, Ashstead, Kent. Has a register of doctors and dentists who are also qualified hypnotherapists. Can also suggest some who have an interest in childbirth.

Association of Post Natal Illnesses, 25 Jerdan Place, London SW6 (tel. 0171 386 0868). Support and advice over the phone (and on a face-to-face basis if the contact lives near to you) for women suffering from all degrees of postnatal illness, given by those who have recovered from it but know how you feel from personal experience. Will also answer letters and offer a good range of helpful leaflets and other literature.

Association of Reflexologists, 27 Old Gloucester Street, London WC1N 3XX.

Avon Episiotomy Support Group, (tel. 0181 482 1453). Nationwide organization offering help, advice and support for women who have had problems with their episiotomy.

John Bell & Croydon, 50 Wigmore Street, London W1H 0AU (tel. 0171 935 5555).

The Birth Centre, 37 Coverton Road, London SW17 (tel. 0171 498 2322). The future trend for part of the independant midwifery service may be towards establishing birth centres. These are specially designed houses which offer facilties such as water pools in private birthing rooms for women who do not wish to give birth at home but would like a more intimate and relaxed environment than a hospital offers. The Birth Centre (located in south London, next to

St George's Hospital) was the first, though others are now
following. It is staffed by independent midwives who can look
after women from all over London, Surrey, Kent and North
Sussex.

Birth Crises, (tel. 0734 698275). Countrywide befriending and
counselling network of mothers trained by birth educator
and author Sheila Kitzinger; will help women who have had
distressing experiences in childbirth. Contact is usually by
phone but can arrange face-to-face counselling, distance
permitting.

BLISS (Baby Life Support Systems), 17–21 Emerald Street,
London WC1 (tel. 0171 831 9393). For parents whose
babies need special care, either because they were premature,
or because they were unwell at birth or soon after they had
been born and needed intensive care in hospital. Support by
phone or face to face; plus helpful literature in the form of
leaflets and books.

Body Treats Aromatherapy Oils, 15 Approach Road, London
SW20 (tel. 0181 543 6333). Good quality oils (also used
by professional aromatherapists) available by mail order.

British Association for Autogenic Training and Therapy, 18
Holtsmere Close, Watford, Herts (letters only) c/o Jane Bird.
Can send you information on AT and put you in touch with
a properly qualified therapist in your area.

British Chiropractic Association, Equity House, 29 Whitely
Street, Reading RG2 O89 (tel. 0134 55557). Can put you in
touch with a professionally qualified practitioner and may
suggest some in your area who have a special interest in
pregnancy, childbirth and postnatal back problems or their
prevention.

British College of Naturopathy and Osteopathy, 6 Netherall
Gardens, London NW3 (tel. 0171 435 6464). Can see
pregnant women for postnatal back problems on any day of
the week, under similar arrangements to the British School of
Osteopathy.

British Homeopathic Association, 2a Devonshire Street,
London W1N IJR (tel. 0171 935 2163). Contact them for a

list of homeopaths who are also medically qualified doctors. If you would prefer a non-medically qualified homeopath, contact the Society of Homeopaths or the Hahnemann Society.

British School of Osteopathy, 1–4 Suffolk Street, London SW1 (0171 930 9254). Holds twice-weekly antenatal and postnatal back clinics to treat any postural problems and back/neck/shoulder pain which have developed as a result of pregnancy, and to prevent such problems from happening in the first place. You will be seen by a senior student, under the strict supervision of an experienced osteopath tutor. Charges are low: about £15 for a first visit and £11 for subsequent visits, compared with the more usual £35 for a first visit with an ordinary osteopath. Their senior tutor Stephen Sandler also teaches specific single-session massage for labour classes.

British Society for Experimental and Clinical Hypnosis, c/o Dr Michael Heap, Dept Psychiatry, The Royal Hallamshire Hospital, Sheffield (tel. 0114 2766222). The society has only qualified health workers in the relevant professions – doctors, midwives, dentists, psychotherapists and psychiatrists – as members. All would be qualified to teach self-hypnosis as a deep relaxation method.

British Wheel of Yoga, 1 Hamilton Place, Boston Road, Sleaford, Lincs (tel. 01529 306 851). Can put you in touch with a professionally qualified teacher near you. Most teachers are happy to have pregnant women in their class if they have done yoga before, and many others will take beginners as long as your GP has said that yoga should be safe for you. Active Birth classes also teach several different yoga exercises for pregnancy and childbirth.

Caesarean Support Network, c/o Yvonne Williams, 55 Cooil Drive, Douglas, Isle of Man (tel. 014624 661269), *or* Sheila Tunstall, 2 Hurst Park Drive, Huyton, Liverpool (tel. 0151 480 1184). Non-medical advice, practical advice and support (both over the phone, and if possible, face to face) on all aspects of caesarean section, from emotional reactions to pain relief: helpful exercises, how to do everything from changing your baby to feeding them the most comfortable way. Plus support and advice for women who would like to try for a vaginal birth after a previous caesarean.

Community Health Councils: see your local telephone directory under C. They have information on all aspects of health care in your area, including maternity care and the practises of different hospitals.

Council of Acupuncture, 19 Gloucester Place, London NW1 (tel. 0171 724 5756). Umbrella body which can put you in touch with a professionally qualified acupuncturist in your area.

Cry-Sis, (tel. 0171 404 5011). National helpline offering support and practical advice for parents of babies who cry excessively, have colic, or sleep badly. The counsellors are all parents who have had, and solved, similar difficulties with their own babies. Also offers useful literature.

Family Planning Association, 27–35 Mortimer Street, London W1 (tel. 0171 636 7866). Runs a helpline Monday to Friday during working hours, which offers confidential advice on sexual and contraceptive problems, including those issues which may arise as a result of childbirth.

General and Registered Council of Osteopaths, 56 London Street, Reading, Berkshire (tel. 0134 56585). Can put you in touch with your nearest qualified osteopath, and may also be able to suggest one or two in your area who have a special interest in pregnancy and the back problems which may follow.

Gingerbread, 35 Wellington Street, London WC2 (tel. 0171 240 0953). Self-help and support groups, advice and information for single parents and their children.

Hahnemann Society, (tel. 0171 837 3297). Contact them for details of non-medically qualified homeopaths.

Health Rights, Unit 405, Brixton Small Business Centre, 444 Brixton Road, London SW9 (tel. 0171 274 4000). Research and advice on all aspects of healthcare – maternity care in particular. Free information by post, or phone.

Helios Homeopathic Pharmacy, (tel. 01892 536 393).
Helpful, knowledgeable staff, rapid mail order service offering
homeopathic tinctures, pills, granules and powders. Will make
up preparations to order.

Incontinence Information Helpline, 'The Helpline', c/o The
Dene Centre, Castle Farm Road, Newcastle-on-Tyne, NE3
1PH (tel. 0191 231 0050). Helpline run by trained nurse
counsellors who can advise you, in total confidence, about
the best way to tackle any continence problems you may have.
(9 a.m.–6 p.m.)

Independent Midwives Association (tel. 01703 694429).
Independent midwives are all trained professionals who have
formerly worked in the NHS and are now practising outside
it. They attend home births, are very supportive of active
and natural birthing practices and so offer great flexibility in
their approach to childbirth. They work on a private basis
and costs for full antenatal, birth and postnatal care including
blood tests and a scan vary widely from around £1,500 to
£2,800 all in. Pain relief options include Entonox, pethidine,
water, TENS, massage. Most have arrangements (called an
Honorary Contract) with their local hospitals, so that if it is
necessary to transfer you to hospital during labour, they will
continue to care for you there too.

Institute of Complementary Medicine, PO Box 194, London
SE16 1QZ (tel. 0171 237 5165). Can supply an extensive
(though not exhaustive) list of qualified complementary
therapists of all types, countrywide.

La Leche League Great Britain, BM3424 London WC1N 3XX
(tel. 0171 242 1278. Offers encouragement, information,
regular group meetings and support (both on the phone and,
distance permitting, in person) for breastfeeding mothers with
all types of breastfeeding problems, including pain. Has large
list of helpful literature, and some useful products associated
with breastfeeding comfort including hypoallergenic lanolin
cream.

MAMA (Meet A Mum Association), 14 Willes Road,
Croydon CRO 2XX (tel. 0181 665 0357). Countrywide

network of self-help and support groups which meet regularly for new mothers to make contact with others in their area.

Maternity Alliance, 59–61 Camden High Street, London NW1 (tel. 0171 837 1265). Campaigns for improvements in social and financial support for pregnant women, and mothers with babies. Will supply information and advice on healthcare, legal rights, and financial support systems available.

Medcare, 39 Ashness Road, Battersea, London SW11. Hire TENS machines out, from about £25 for four weeks.

Medical Advisory Service, (tel. 0181 995 8503). Nationwide helpline staffed by ex-NHS trained nurse counsellors, who can offer advice and refer you on to the relevant support or helplines on any medical issue, including those which can arise as a result of childbirth.

National Childbirth Trust, Alexandra House, Oldham Terrace, London W3 (tel. 0171 992 8637). Advice, help and support on all aspects of pregnancy, childbirth and breastfeeding. Will (where distance permits) visit breastfeeding mothers who are experiencing difficulties and also offer telephone help. Groups and classes nationwide. Large range of useful books and leaflets on everything from becoming a father and vaginal birth after a caesarean, to breastfeeding a toddler and home birth. NCT Maternity Sales on 0141 633 5552 offer a catalogue of items catering for the needs of pregnant and breastfeeding women, including a good range of feeding bras and breast pumps.

National Institute of Medical Herbalists, 9 Palace Gate, Exeter, Devon EX1 IJA (tel. 01392 426 022). Traditional herbs can be extremely useful for encouraging post childbirth recovery in general, and for helping certain types of painful problem after labour – especially helping tears and episiotomy sites to heal rapidly. The Institute can put you in touch with a qualified herbalist in your area.

Neals Yard Remedies, 14–15 Neals Yard, London WC2 (tel. 0171 379 0705). Chain of shops selling good quality aromatherapy oils, herbs, Bach flower remedies, basic homeopathic preparations and natural ointments. Staff are usually helpful and knowledgable. Mail order service and enquiries to the address above.

Positively Women, (tel. 0171 490 5575). An organization run by women, for women who are HIV positive or who have AIDS. Can advise on some of the issues surrounding pregnancy and birth if you are HIV positive, and refer you on to other expert sources of relevant information. Also runs help groups, counselling service and support groups.

Pre-eclampsia Society, 1 South Avenue, Hullbridge, Hockley, Southend, Essex. Nationwide network of help groups offering support for women with pre-eclampsia, plus advice and information on its management and causes. Regular newsletter and helpful literature.

Research Council for Complementary Medicine, 60 Great Ormond Street, London WC1 (tel. 0171 833 8897). Contact this organization if you would like to follow up a particular aspect of the use of complementary medicine for childbirth – either for your own information or to use as ammunition for any discussions with medical staff who do not seem to be well disposed to the idea of you using complementary therapies to help you during labour. They have a large, though incomplete, database of clinical trials and information on the clinical usage of all the therapies. There is a small charge for access to this information.

Royal College of Midwives, 15 Mansfield Street, London W1 (tel. 0171 637 8823). Can advise on all aspects of midwifery practice in Britain. Will know of many of the departments of midwifery in hospitals countrywide who have a particular interest in or symapthy for different ways of giving birth and providing pain relief. Also if you are having difficulty with your local hospital because you are most anxious to have a particular type of pain relief and the unit is unhappy about it, the RCM could advise you.

Royal College of Obstetricians, 27 Sussex Place, Regents Park, London NW1 (tel. 0171 262 5425). Has a helpline service which can answer queries on all aspects of pregnancy and childbirth.

Society of Homeopaths, (tel. 01604 21400). Contact them for details of non-medically qualified homeopaths.

Splashdown, 1 Wellington Terrace, Harrow on the Hill, Middlesex (tel. 0181 422 9308). Rents and delivers birthing pools for use at home, or in hospital. Prices at the time of writing from about £150.

Twins and Multiple Births Association, 59 Sunnyside, Worksop, Nottinghamshire (tel. 01732 868000). Advice on all aspects of pregnancy, birth and looking after twins (or more). Helpline operates from 6 p.m.–11 p.m. weekdays only.

Glossary

Acupuncture An ancient Chinese form of medicine involving the insertion of fine needles into different parts of the body to treat illness, and soothe pain.

After pains Contractions of the uterus which occur after the baby has been born. They may be felt as a sensation, some women experience them as pain, others notice nothing at all.

Anaesthesia The use of chemical agents to render someone unconscious. This is sometimes used in obstetrics for emergency caesarean sections.

Analgesia Pain relief. It may be a drug or a non-pharmacological method.

Areola The pigmented area of the breast on the flat part around the nipple.

Aromatherapy The use of essential oils of plants thought to encourage the release of various neurochemicals in the body for pain-relieving, relaxing, and healing purposes.

Assisted delivery Medical intervention to help the baby out of the birth canal, either with forceps or ventouse suction.

Autogenic training Deep relaxation therapy aimed at relieving stress, which can be used for reducing pain in labour.

Birth canal The unified passage of the uterus, the dilated cervix and the vagina along which the baby passes in birth. It is only present as an open canal during the second stage of labour.

Bradykinin An enzyme made in the tissues during muscle damage which irritates the nerve endings.

Braxton-Hicks' contractions During pregnancy the uterus is making mild contractions, limbering up and getting ready for labour. These are felt by different women to different degrees, but they are not labour contractions and are not associated with dilation of the cervix.

Breast abscess A collection of pus similar to a boil which occasionally develops in the breast. This needs medical treatment, possibly incising and drainage.

Breathing and relaxation A natural form of relaxation used for pain relief in labour. You need to practise it as often as possible antenatally to get the best effect.

Breech delivery When the baby presents itself bottom rather than head first. A breech delivery is a little more difficult to manage than is a head-first one and demands greater skill from the midwifery and medical staff.

Bromocriptine A hormone used if milk production should become excessive or if it is necessary to suppress lactation. It is given under medical prescription.

Bupivacaine A local anaesthetic used in epidural anaesthesia.

Caesarean section Delivery of the baby via an incision in the mother's abdomen and uterus. It can be done under general anaesthetic, but more usually done with epidural or spinal anaesthesia.

Catecholamines Hormones produced in the adrenal gland and other parts of the body which transport pain signals and cause contractions of the uterus. They are usually secreted in the second stage of labour, and encourage the strong, expulsive contractions of the womb which are needed at this time.

Cephalopelvic disproportion When the baby's head is too large to pass easily through the woman's bony pelvis. It may be because of the baby having a very big head, because the head is incorrectly flexed, or because the mother has a smaller than average pelvis.

Cervix The neck of the womb. In the non-pregnant state it is almost closed, leaving a canal only a millimetre or two in diameter which allows menstrual blood to escape each month. Once pregnancy starts, the cervix keeps the baby in the uterus. During labour it dilates to 10cm to allow the passage of the baby down the birth canal.

Colporrhapy A repair operation on the vaginal muscles and lining.

Congenital abnormalities Sometimes during the early days of formation of the embryo, certain fetal parts do not develop perfectly, producing an abnormality. A few of these are serious, eg those of the heart, brain or spinal cord. But most, such as extra fingers or toes are not life-threatening.

Contractions The flexing of the uterus muscles in labour.

Cortisol A hormone made by the adrenal gland which helps the body deal with stress.

Couvade The way in which some male partners may feel sympathetic labour pains when their partner is in childbirth.

Dura The outer covering of the membrane sac containing the spinal fluid, the spinal cord and its nerves.

Eclampsia When the mother experiences fits during her pregnancy/ labour. Usually associated with raised blood pressure and protein in the urine.

Endorphins Naturally produced morphine-like substances made in the brain which help block pain.

Engorgement of breasts Milk is made in the glandular tissue of the breasts and passes into the ducts for storage. Sometimes the production exceeds demand and the breasts become engorged or swollen. *Primary engorgement* follows the increase in fluid at the beginning of milk production in the first two to three days after delivery. This usually settles when the baby becomes more used to the habit of feeding and takes milk easily from the breast. *Secondary engorgement* may come later, when, after having fed the baby for a while, there may be a build-up of the milk in some part or in the whole of the breast. It could develop into an inflammation, and would need attention to prevent this.

Entonox Form of pain relief consisting of a pre-mixed cylinder of fifty-fifty nitrous oxide and oxygen.

Epidural anaesthetic A local anaesthetic introduced to the tissues around the spinal sac to numb the nerves as they flow back to the spinal cord. It is not a spinal anaesthetic. Usually this means that the woman has to stay in bed because of weakness in the legs, but a fragmented dose can be given in some specialist units so that the she can be mobile in labour. This is called a mobile or ambulant epidural.

Epifoam An anaesthetic foam sprayed on to the perineum after delivery. It contains a mixture of a local anaesthetic and a steroid anti-inflammatory, and is very helpful for soothing painful perineal stitches.

Episiotomy A clean cut made under local anaesthesic in the perineum at the back of the vagina, during a uterine contraction, to make more room for the baby's head to pass through.

Fetal distress This is when the fetus becomes short of oxygen. As it can be dangerous, and it is one common reason for a caesarean section.

Fetal medicine The science of understanding and looking after the fetus (the unborn child).

Fibrosis One way in which the body's tissues heal is by laying down fibrous tissue. These contract (pucker) a little, in the same way that scar tissue sometimes does.

First stage of labour The first stage or part of childbirth is when the uterus is contracting and the neck of the womb (cervix) is opening. During the first stage, the cervix opens up completely to about 10cm wide.

Forceps delivery   Assisted delivery using forceps instrument.

Gas   In the sense of pain relief, this usually refers to nitrous oxide (sometimes called laughing gas). See *Entonox* above.

General anaesthesia   In the United Kingdom, this is now mostly used for some emergency caesarean sections and a few elective caesarean sections. The woman can request a general anaesthetic but, if there is time, and she wishes it, a spinal or an epidural anaesthetic for caesarean section allows her to be awake and with her partner to take part in the delivery.

Granulation   Proud flesh where the inflammatory response continues, even after underlying tissues have healed. This can be painful and may be difficult to treat.

Haematoma   An internal bruise where blood collects in a cavity in the body. This feels like a lump if you run your finger across its surface, and it may be tender to touch.

Haemorrhoids (Piles)   Piles are protrusions of part of the lining of the anal canal filled with veins. They may protrude through the anus after childbirth but usually go back either on their own, or with simple treatments.

Homeopathy   The giving of tiny amounts of natural substances diluted many thousands of times as a remedy for a wide range of conditions.

Hypnotherapy   A process by which a woman is put into a state of deep relaxation (which can help her labour to progress easily). Experienced hypnotherapists can with some people make part of the body numb merely by putting their hand on the area; this is known as *glove hypnosis*. They can also teach women successfully to hypnotize themselves.

Induction   A procedure to start labour such as prostaglandin pessaries or breaking the amniotic membranes.

Ischaemia   Lack of oxygen to the muscles. This may cause an area of muscle to spasm painfully (as in angina) and is one cause of pain in labour.

Labial tears   At delivery small tears of the fleshy lips around the vulva may occur. These may need attention after childbirth but usually heal quickly and easily on their own.

Labour   The process of childbirth. It is the time when the uterus is actively contracting and the neck of the womb opening. The combination of the two allows the baby to pass down the birth canal and be born.

Lactic acid   When muscle cells work, waste products accumulate. One of these is an organic acid known as lactic acid. It has to be washed out of the circulation, broken down into carbon dioxide and breathed out through the lungs. If it is allowed to build up perhaps when muscles are working very hard, such as in a long-distance run or during labour it can make the muscle fibres sore.

Lochia After the baby is born, the uterus expels a little old blood and other tissue for the next few days. This blood-like loss turns slowly pink, then brownish-yellow over the next two weeks, as it tails off.

Marcaine A local anaesthetic used in epidural anaesthesia.

Mastitis An inflammation of the breast which may be non-infective (ie caused by a blocked duct) or infected (due to bacterial infestation). *Recurrent mastitis* occurs when infection does not settle with primary treatment but comes back again after the treatment has stopped.

Meconium The greenish waste substance that fills the large bowel of the baby before they are born. Usually it stays there until after delivery, but if the baby becomes short of oxygen its large bowel may contract while the baby is still in the uterus and push the meconium into the amniotic fluid. This then passes down the vagina and is noted as a greenish staining at the entrance. Meconium is one sign of fetal distress.

Meptazinol A pain-relieving drug.

Morphine A pain-relieving drug related to opium.

Naloxone A stimulant used for the baby if he is not breathing at birth, following depression of respiration for pharmacological reasons.

Natural pain relief The relief of the pain of labour by non-pharmacological methods such as relaxation and breathing or acupuncture.

Nitrous oxide A pain relieving agent (laughing gas) usually given mixed with oxygen. It used to be mixed with air (gas and air) but this stopped in the UK twenty years ago.

Pessary Interim measure to treat prolapse of the womb. A plastic ring which fits around the cervix, holding the womb upwards and back while allowing the cervix to protrude through a hole in the middle, so any menstrual blood can flow out normally.

Oxytocin A hormone produced in the pituitary gland which stimulates the uterus to contract.

Pain threshold The point at which sensory stimuli are perceived as painful. Most people's pain thresholds are similar. It is their tolerance levels which vary.

Pain tolerance The ability of someone to stand pain is their tolerance level. It depends on a wide variety of different physical and psychological factors which affect the way their systems mediate pain – from relaxation or fear to pain-relieving drugs – after the stimulus has passed the threshold level.

Paracervical block Injection of a local anaesthetic agent to the nerves running from the uterus as they pass on either side of the cervix. If used, it would usually be given at the end of the first stage. It is useful for assisted deliveries (such as vacuum or forceps) but is not used now so often in this country, having been replaced by epidural anaesthetic.

Perinatal The time around birth. Conventionally, perinatal as an adjective is used in the United Kingdom from the 24th week of pregnancy until a week after birth.

Perineum This is the muscular area between the opening of the vagina and the rectum. It stretches considerably in front of the baby's head during birth, but may need some suturing afterwards.

Pethidine A strong pain-relieving and sedative drug which is helpful in labour for many women.

Pharmacological pain relief Painkilling drugs which can only be prescribed by qualified medical or midwifery staff.

Placenta praevia If the placenta is implanted low down on the uterus wall, below the baby, it could cause severe bleeding at the time of delivery. This is often diagnosed with ultrasound, and the mother is advised about the method of delivery accordingly.

Placental abruption When the placenta begins to separate from the uterine wall it can result in considerable bleeding. This is a medical emergency which requires urgent action, including an immediate caesarean.

Potency How effective a drug is at various concentrations. Different people have varying responses to drugs, and so may require a higher or lower dosage than the average person. This term is also used to describe the strength of homeopathic preparations.

Pre-eclampsia Continuous raised blood pressure during pregnancy. This may affect the growth of the fetus, resulting in a small baby; it can often be very effectively controlled but may mean admission to hospital during the latter part of pregnancy and a medically managed labour or even a caesarean section. If it becomes severe it can lead to *eclampsia* (see p. 310).

Prolapse The dropping of the uterus down the vagina, which may occur some time after a difficult delivery. Its treatment is mainly by exercises or by surgical procedures. It is also possible to have a prolapse of the rectum or urinary tube after very prolonged pushing in the second stage of labour. These too can be repaired very effectively.

Psychosomatic pain Pain which has no obvious physical cause.

Though its origins may be psychological, it can hurt every bit as much as if it had a physical cause.

Pudendal block   An injection of local anaesthetic into the nerves which supply the perineum to numb it during delivery. Also used for episiotomies.

Reflexology   A form of pain relief using very precise selective, gentle pressure on areas of the hands and feet to help treat disorders, or reduce pain.

Relaxin   A hormone made in the body during pregnancy to help soften the ligaments of the pelvis, so it stretches to offer a passage for the baby.

Sacrosciatac joint   The articulation between the sacrum and the iliac bones of the pelvis. There is one joint on each side, situated under the dimples in the back just above the bottom. The joints loosen a little in pregnancy allowing an easier passage for the baby's head, but this can cause back strain and backache afterwards.

Second stage of labour   The expulsive stage of labour when the woman actively pushes and the baby passes through the birth canal to be born.

Show   The discharge of blood-stained mucus from the vagina – one of the signs of the onset of labour.

Spinal block   An injection of local anaesthetic into the fluid around the spinal cord to numb the lower segments of the nerve. This is not an epidural and is used for caesareans rather than general pain relief in labour.

Third stage of labour   The stage of labour when, after the birth of the baby, the placenta and membranes are delivered.

Transcutaneous Electrical Nerve Stimulation (TENS)   A form of pain relief involving a low-grade electrical current passed through pads, into the skin of the back.

Transverse lie   When the baby is lying across the line of the longitudinal axis of the uterus: perhaps across your abdomen, sideways rather than head-down. It is unlikely the baby can be delivered vaginally because, as uterine contractions start, the baby's back would be folded towards the cervix, preventing it from passing through. A persistent transverse lie which cannot be altered (some obstetricians have used manual massage of the mother's abdomen to encourage her baby to turn around into the correct position) means a caesarean section is necessary.

Ultrasound   A method of looking at the fetus while it is in the uterus, using sound waves.

Uterus   The uterus (womb) is the muscular organ that contains the growing baby. For 38 weeks it stretches from the size and shape of a very small pear to that of a large watermelon so that the baby can grow from a few cells into a separate person. Also in the uterus are the placenta and the amniotic fluid. During labour the uterine muscle contracts to expel the baby.

Vacuum delivery   Assisted delivery using a vacuum-suction device.

Vulva   The vulva is the area guarding the vagina from the outside world. It consists of two fleshy lips on the outer surface which bear hair. Inside these are two finer lips which are not hair-bearing. Normally these are held together to protect the vagina from infection.

Zylocaine   A local anaesthetic used to relieve pain in the perineum when an episiotomy is being done.

Index